MEDICAL BOARDS STEP 1
made ridiculously simple

Andreas Carl, M.D., Ph.D.
Research Assistant Professor
University of Nevada Reno
School of Medicine
Department of Physiology and Cell Biology
Reno, NV 89557-0046

MedMaster, Inc., Miami

ISBN #0-940780-25-9

Made in the United States of America

Published by
MedMaster, Inc.
P.O. Box 640028
Miami, FL 33164

For Dr. Anna Ivanenko.

This project would not have been possible without her
encouragement and enthusiasm.

INTRODUCTION

What kind of score you will get on the USMLE Step 1 exam does not only depend on how hard you study, but also on what you study. Obviously, if you study what they ask, you will achieve a very high score. I have prepared this manuscript in order to help you to maximize your efforts. The material has been selected based on several years of teaching basic medical sciences to medical students and my own recent experience with the USMLE Step 1. It has worked very well for me and I hope will do the same for you.

These tables do not replace any textbooks. They are designed to provide you with a "core knowledge" that should be memorized as well as possible. I have chosen the table-format in order to provide the maximum amount of information with the minimum amount of words. I believe that this format facilitates memorization. By concentrating on the key associations you will certainly improve your performance in "multiple choice situations".

How to use these tables: I recommend reviewing the tables many times until they become boring. This is a good sign - meaning you recognize the stuff. It's probably not necessary to be able to actively reproduce the material given here (although it wouldn't hurt), as long as you recognize the key associations in a "multiple choice situation". I have tried to be comprehensive but brief. You will find most of the material very simplified, perhaps oversimplified and often you may find it necessary to consult your textbooks, in order to make sense out of it. As you become familiar with the material and increasingly bored, you should be able to read through these tables within a couple of hours and still maintain a relaxed state of mind - now you are ready to take the USMLE Step 1 exam!

A few words about selection of this material: You will find Anatomy, Social Sciences and Physiology under represented and Pathology somewhat over represented here. Anatomy has been kept short because a) it's highly visual, you profit more by looking at the pictures in an atlas, rather than reading words, b) there have been only few Anatomy questions on recent USMLE Step 1 exams. Social Sciences and Physiology are under represented since they are conceptual sciences and contain only a small amount of hard core facts. You need to be aware that for these two subjects knowing only the tables given here is not sufficient to bring you a good score. This is particularly true for Physiology! I have over emphasized Pathology somewhat, because I believe it is the most useful of the basic sciences for your future career and will be an invaluable help for studying of Internal Medicine in the 3rd and 4th years of Medical School.

I thank Steve Goldberg for the cartoons. Figures 4.23-4.32 were modified and reproduced with permission from Smith, L.H. and Thier, S.O. *Pathophysiology - The Biological Principles of Disease*. W.D. Saunders Co., 1985.

I hope that this text will help your preparation for the USMLE Step 1 and would appreciate any comments about the selection and presentation of this material you might have.

Good luck!

PATHOLOGY

- This should be the center piece of your studies, it's also the most valuable for your future practice.

- I prefer Rubin and Farber's Pathology (14) over Robbins-Cotran (15) as a primary text book because of its incredibly beautiful illustrations.

- Spend a full week just looking at pictures, until you can distinguish a papillary thyroid carcinoma from a follicular one (with closed eyes, in the middle of the night and blind - just kidding).

- If you are ambitious, go over Compton's Review Questions (16). These are very difficult ! If you get about 50% right, you should do very well on the Boards.

MICROBIOLOGY

- Just study them bug by bug, Levinson-Jawetz, (13) is an excellent text.

- Also check out *Clinical Microbiology Made Ridiculously Simple* (6). This book contains over 200 cartoons which makes microbiology much more digestible.

- Know all the details, structure/function of the HIV virus. Study therapy of AIDS related infectious diseases.

- If you have time to spare, read "Immunology" from the NMS series (12). There are many questions on the exam, and this book covers it all.

PHARMACOLOGY

- Harvey-Champe (18) is "dead-on". If you know this book, you should get close to 100% right.

- *Clinical Pharmacology Made Ridiculously Simple* (8) contains a large number of tables comparing drugs side by side. Very complete! Excellent review, not just for the Boards but also for later.

- I found flash cards very useful. Make two sets : One for drug names vs. mechanism of action and/or indication, and one set for drug names vs. side effects.

BIOCHEMISTRY

- Champe-Harvey (2) is "dead-on". If you know this book, you should get close to 100% right.

- In case you got lost, I recommend *Clinical Biochemistry Made Ridiculously Simple* (5) for a quick overview of the wondrous and amazing Land of Biochemistry.

ANATOMY

- Don't spend too much time on this subject. Best preparation is to look at pictures, including plenty of cross sections (CT or MRI scans) of the body.

- Read *Clinical Anatomy Made Ridiculously Simple* (4), but even this may be overkill.

- Read *Clinical Neuroanatomy Made Ridiculously Simple* (7). Read this one twice !

- Make sure you know basic Embryology to get some easy points.

PHYSIOLOGY

- Most difficult subject, cause you can't memorize it. Even if you knew your Ganong (20) or Guyton (23) 100%, you won't be able to answer all questions. If you had lots of time (which you don't) you might consider Best & Taylors *Physiological Basis of Medical Practice* (19). I like Despopoulos-Silbernagel *Color Atlas of Physiology* (8) for quick review.

- Concentrate on kidney, heart and lung !

- A recent trend on the Boards is receptors, signal transduction mechanisms and molecular biology of the cell.

- Make sure you can calculate renal clearance without getting a panic attack!

SOCIAL SCIENCES

- Don't waste too much time here, but read *Behavioral Science for the Boreds* (1). Some things you need to know very well are :

- Differences between normal grief reaction and adjustment disorders, neuroses and psychoses, dementia and delirium.

- Defense mechanisms.

- Sensitivity / Specificity / Negative predictive value etc. It's not enough to memorize what to divide by what, you need to understand the meaning of these.

- Design of clinical trials.

PRETEST SERIES

- I found the *Pretest Questions* similar in style but slightly more difficult than the actual board exam. The Appleton & Lange questions (21) are a bit easier and excellent for review. Don't use these questions to "test" yourself. Mark wrong answers, identify your areas of weakness and concentrate your studies on these.

TEST TAKING STRATEGIES

- Don't practice multiple choice questions the week before the exam. You will get tired, bored and frustrated. Negative feelings will then carry over to the exam day.

- Don't study any new material the day before the exam.

- If you can't even guess a question, choose either the longest answer or the one that is most similar to other choices. Then move on. Don't be upset, this happens a lot and is quite normal. If you have the feeling you might be able to answer it if you could only think hard enough, skip it and come back to it if time allows.

- Make sure you time yourself very well. I found it useful to answer questions in blocks of 15. This actually saves some time and you get little breaks marking the sheet.

- Don't eat a heavy lunch! Good luck!

REFERENCES

1. Behavioral Science for the Boreds, F.S. Sierles, MedMaster Inc.
2. Biochemistry, Champe-Harvey, Lippincott
3. Biochemistry, Stryer, Freeman
4. Clinical Anatomy Made Ridiculously Simple, S.Goldberg, MedMaster Inc.
5. Clinical Biochemistry Made Ridiculously Simple, S.Goldberg, MedMaster Inc.
6. Clinical Microbiology Made Ridiculously Simple, Gladwin-Trattler, MedMaster Inc.
7. Clinical Neuroanatomy Made Ridiculously Simple, S.Goldberg, MedMaster Inc.
8. Clinical Pharmacology Made Ridiculously Simple, J. Olson, MedMaster Inc.
9. Color-Atlas of Physiology, Despopoulos-Silbernagl, Thieme
10. Comprehensive Textbook of Psychiatry, Kaplan, Williams & Wilkin
11. Drug Evaluations, American Medical Association
12. Immunology, R.Hyde, Harwal Publishing
13. Medical Microbiology & Immunology, Levinson-Jawetz, Appleton & Lange
14. Pathology, Rubin & Farber, Lippincott
15. Pathologic Basis of Disease, Robbins-Cotran, Saunders
16. Pathologic Basis of Disease - Selfassessment and Review, Saunders
17. Pharmacologic Basis of Therapeutics, Goodman & Gilman, Macmillan
18. Pharmacology, Harvey-Champe, Lippincott
19. Physiological Basis of Medical Practice, J.B.West, Williams & Wilkin
20. Review of Medical Physiology, W.F. Ganong, Appleton&Lange
21. Review for National Boards Part 1, M.Caplan, Appleton & Lange
22. Sherris Medical Microbiology, K.J. Ryan, Appleton & Lange
23. Textbook of Medical Physiology, Guyton, Saunders

TABLE OF CONTENT

1. PATHOLOGY

2. MICROBIOLOGY

3. PHARMACOLOGY

4. BIOCHEMISTRY

5. ANATOMY

6. PHYSIOLOGY

7. SOCIAL SCIENCE

8. ABBREVIATIONS

PATHOLOGY

USMLE Step 1
Pathology

25. The specimen below:
   - A. Is poorly fixed
   - B. Is poorly photographed
   - C. Shows some sort of disease
   - D. All of the above

1.1.) <u>AUTOSOMAL RECESSIVE DISORDERS</u>

cystic fibrosis	pulmonary infections, diabetes
phenylketonuria	light skin, mental retardation
albinism	sunburn, skin cancer
α1-antitrypsin deficiency	COPD, liver cirrhosis
thalassemias, sickle cell anemias	anemia
glycogen storage diseases	liver, muscle, heart
mucopolysaccharidoses (except Hunter's)	facial deformities, mental and physical retardation
sphingolipidoses (except Fabry's)	hepatomegaly, splenomegaly etc.
polycystic renal disease (infant type)	kidney failure
hemochromatosis	liver cirrhosis
Chediak-Higashi	bacterial infections due to impaired neutrophil chemotaxis

1.2.) <u>AUTOSOMAL DOMINANT DISORDERS</u>

familial hypercholesterolemia	ischemic heart disease
familial polyposis	colon cancer
spherocytosis	hemolytic anemia
Von Willebrand	bleeding
Ehlers Danlos	stretchy skin sprains, joint dislocations
Marfan's	long bones lens dislocation
achondroplasia	premature ossification dwarfism
phacomatoses	benign tumors of eye, skin and brain
Huntington's	chorea dementia
polycystic renal disease (adult type)	kidney failure a/w berry aneurysms

1.3.) <u>X-LINKED RECESSIVE DISORDERS</u>

hemophilia A and B	bleeding
glucose-6-phosphate def.	hemolytic anemia
fragile X	mental retardation
Fabry's	angiokeratoma cardiomegaly
Lesch-Nyhan	self mutilation gout
Duchenne, Becker's	muscle dystrophy
Bruton's (agammaglobulinemia)	B cell defect
Wiskott-Aldrich	B cell and T cells defects thrombocytopenia
chronic granulomatous disease	defect in neutrophil free radical formation bacterial infections

1.4.) <u>MOST COMMON CAUSES</u>

cancer in man[1]	**lung** > prostate > colon
cancer in woman[1]	**breast** > colon > lung
cancer in children	leukemia (ALL)

[1] Incidence except skin cancer. For mortality see table 7.1.

acute renal failure	tubular necrosis
nephrotic syndrome	children : minimal change glomerulonephritis
	adults : membranous glomerulonephritis
nephritic syndrome	poststreptococcal glomerulonephritis
hypertension	"idiopathic" > renal
anemia	iron deficiency
amenorrhea	pregnancy
chronic pancreatitis	alcoholism
food poisoning	Clostridia perfringens
	Staph.aureus toxin

1.5.) MOST COMMON INFECTIVE CAUSES

common cold	rhino viruses
pharyngitis, laryngitis	viral > bacterial (ß-hemolysing Strept.)
tonsillitis	ß-hemolysing Strept.
sinusitis	Strep.pneumoniae, Staph.aureus
otitis media	Strep.pneumoniae, Hemophilus influenza
bronchitis	Hemophilus influenza, Strep.pneumoniae
pneumonia	Influenza A virus > Strept.pneumoniae
meningitis - neonates **- infants** **- adults** **- elderly** **- overall**	**Strep. agalactia, E.coli** **Hemophilus influenza** **Neisseria meningitidis** **Strep. pneumoniae** **Hemophilus influenza**
encephalitis	viral
endocarditis	Strep.viridans
post transfusion hepatitis	hepatitis C
carbuncle	Staph.aureus
sepsis (catheterized patient)	Staph.aureus, Candida
sepsis (burn wounds)	Pseudomonas aeruginosa
diarrhea - children **- adult (US)** **- traveler**	**rota virus** **Campylobacter** **E.coli, shigella, salmonella**
genital ulcer	herpes > syphilis
urethritis	chlamydia > gonococcus
cystitis	E.coli

1.6.) <u>HYPERSENSITIVITY</u>

Type I	IgE mast cells basophils	urticaria erythema bronchiole constr. laryngeal edema shock, death	**asthma** hay fever eczema
Type II	**IgM, IgG** antibody dependent cell mediated cytotoxicity	hemolysis	**transfusion reaction** drug reactions erythroblastosis fetalis autoimmune diseases[1]
Type III	**IgM, IgG** immune complexes	urticaria lymphadenopathy arthritis vasculitis glomerulonephritis	**serum sickness** Arthus reaction
Type IV	"delayed hypersensitivity" **T cell** mediated (memory cells)	erythema with induration	**tuberculin reaction**

Transplant rejection
hyperacute   *due to preformed antibodies*
   acute   *involves type I and type IV mechanisms*

[1] examples :

rheumatoid arthritis	anti IgG
systemic lupus	anti ds DNA
myasthenia gravis	anti ACh receptor
Graves disease	anti TSH receptor
Wegener's granulomatosis	anti neutrophil cytoplasmic (ANCA)

1.7.) <u>SLE</u>

ANA	:	most sensitive
anti dsDNA and anti-sm	:	most specific
LE cell	:	nucleus from artificially injured leukocyte being phagocytized

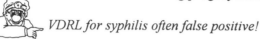 *VDRL for syphilis often false positive!*

1.8.) <u>SCLERODERMA & SJÖGREN'S</u>

Scleroderma	Sjögren's
- limited = CREST - diffuse systemic	- dry eyes, dry mouth
- **anti centromere** - **anti Scl-70** (topoisomerase I)	- **SS-A** (anti Ro) - **SS-B** (anti La)

1.9.) <u>AMYLOID</u>

AL	:	Amyloid light chains
AA	:	Amyloid associated protein

a/w aging, rheumatoid arthritis, inflammatory bowel disease, multiple myeloma and many more.

1.10.) <u>TUMOR MARKERS</u>

AFP	:	hepatoma, twin pregnancy, anencephalus
CEA	:	colon CA, pancreas CA
HCG	:	choriocarcinoma, hydatiform mole, germinoma

Acid phosphatase	:	prostate
Alkaline phosphatase	:	bone, liver, leukemia

1.11.) IMMUNODEFICIENCIES

severe combined	lymphoid stem cells	X-linked or autosomal	death within first year
DiGeorge's	T cells absent	sporadic	viral infections fungal infections tetany
Bruton's	B cells absent	X-linked	bacterial infections
common variable	B cells present but produce little Ab	variable	bacterial infections
IgA deficiency	low IgA	autosomal	sinupulmonary infections gastrointestinal infections
Wiscott Aldrich	low IgM	X-recessive	bacterial infections thrombocytopenia eczema

most common congenital immunodeficiency : IgA deficiency
most common acquired immunodeficiency   : AIDS

1.12.) __BLEEDING DISORDERS__

idiopathic thrombocytic purpura	- immune mediated - acute (viral inf. children) - chronic (adults)
thrombotic thrombocytic purpura	- young woman - microthrombi - fragmented RBCs (helmet cells)
factor VIII-R (Von Willebrand)	- **PTT** prolonged - **bleeding time** prolonged
factor VIII (hemophilia A)	- **PTT** prolonged - normal bleeding time
factor IX (hemophilia B)	- **PTT** prolonged - normal bleeding time
Vit. K (II, V, VII, IX, X)	- fat malabsorption - antibiotics (gut flora) - coumarins

Bleeding Time : platelet function
PT :   extrinsic + common pathways
PTT :   intrinsic + common pathways
TT :   common pathway

1.13.) <u>HEMOLYTIC ANEMIAS</u>

spherocytosis	- auto-dominant - defective spectrin - splenomegaly

G6PD	- hemolysis during oxidative stress such as:
	    viral infections, fava beans,
	      sulfa drugs, quinine, nitrofurantoin
	- Heinz bodies (hemoglobin degradation products)

sickle cells	- **HbS** $(\alpha_2\beta^s_2)$ - hypoxia, dehydration, low pH - vaso-occlusive crisis - aplastic crisis - sequestration crisis (splenomegaly) - autosplenectomy
α-Thalassemias	- **HbH** (β_4) - **Hb Barts** (γ_4), hydrops fetalis - hypochromic cells
β-Thalassemias[1]	- **HbA$_2$** $(\alpha_2\delta_2)$ and **HbF** $(\alpha_2\gamma_2)$ - hypochromic cells

autoimmune	- **warm antibodies : IgG**
	    (drugs, malignancy, SLE)
	- **cold antibodies : IgM**
	    (mycoplasma, mononucleosis, lymphoma)
	
	- Coombs test positive (direct/indirect)[2]

[1]**major** : homozygote,   **minor** : heterozygote

[2]**direct** : cell bound Ab,   **indirect** : free Ab

1.14.) OTHER ANEMIAS

megaloblastic	- hypochromic, macrocytic - hypersegmented neutrophils - folate : anemia, no neurological symptoms - B12 : anemia plus neurological symptoms

iron deficiency	- hypochromic, microcytic
	- blood loss
	- Plummer-Vinson : anemia
	                          atrophic glossitis
	                          esophageal webs

aplastic	- congenital (= Fanconi's) - infections - drugs : alkylating agents chloramphenicol

1.15.) <u>RED BLOOD CELLS</u>

Heinz bodies	- G6PD deficiency - denatured hemoglobin
Howell-Jolly bodies	- post splenectomy - nuclear fragments
basophil stippling	- lead poisoning
siderocytes	- iron overload - Pappenheimer bodies
reticulocytes	- increased production of RBC - a/w hemorrhage - RNA

1.16.) NEUTROPENIA

decreased production	- megaloblastic anemia - some leukemias, lymphomas
increased destruction	- immune mediated (e.g. Felty's)
drug induced	- alkylating agents - chloramphenicol - chlorpromazine - sulfonamides - phenylbutazone

1.17.) LEUKOCYTOSIS

PMN leukocytosis	- acute infections - stress
eosinophilic leukocytosis	- allergy, asthma - parasitic infections
lymphocytosis	- tuberculosis - viral infections
monocytosis	- tuberculosis - malaria - rickettsia

1.18.) LEUKEMIA

ALL	AML	CML	CLL	Hairy cells
fever petechiae ecchymoses CNS infiltrate	fever petechiae ecchymoses lymphadenopathy (splenomegaly)	fever night sweats splenomegaly	insidious few symptoms low Ig levels infections	hepatomegaly splenomegaly TRAP
prognosis : fair	**poor**	**poor**	**fair**	**poor**
lymphoblasts	Auer rods in myeloblasts	Philadelphia chr. (22 -> 9) in myeloid stem cells	lymphocytes predominate	pancytopenia hairy cells in bone marrow

15

1.19.) <u>LYMPHOMA</u>

Hodgkin	Non-Hodgkin (NHL)
- spread in contiguity - no leukemic component - Reed-Sternberg cells	- do not spread in contiguity - often have leukemic component

<u>Subclassifications :</u>

Hodgkin	- lymphocyte predominance - nodular sclerosis	better prognosis
	- mixed cellularity - lymphocyte depletion	many Reed Sternberg cells = poor prognosis
NHL	- nodular or diffuse	-
	- lymphocytic, mixed or <u>histiocytic</u>	-
	-<u>lymphoblastic</u> or undifferentiated (=**Burkitt's**)	- "starry sky" pattern[1]

Note : underlined ones have <u>poorest</u> prognosis

[1] *the "stars" : benign macrophages*
    the "sky"   : matrix of rapidly proliferating neoplastic B cells

Cutaneous T cell lymphomas : mycosis fungoides and **Sézary**

1.20.) PLASMA CELL NEOPLASIA

Multiple Myeloma	Waldenström's	Monoclonal Gammopathy
malignant **IgG type, IgA type etc.**	malignant **IgM**	benign ("early disease" ?)
Bence Jones Proteins (free light chains)	Bence Jones P. in only 10%	M-proteins
"myeloma cells" (plasma cells which infiltrate BM) Russell's bodies Osteoclast activating factor ("punched out" skull, pelvis, etc.)	"flame cells" (eosinophilic plasma cells)	

1.21.) <u>PHLEBOTHROMBOSIS</u>

- bluish red, without lines of Zahn

  - **Virchow's triad** :　　　- endothelial injury
  　　　　　　　　　　　　 - slow blood flow
  　　　　　　　　　　　　 - hypercoagulability

  - **Trousseau's sign** :　　 - migratory venous thrombosis
  　　　　　　　　　　　　 - a/w neoplasms

1.22.) <u>ARTERIOSCLEROSIS</u>

atherosclerosis	- large and medium size arteries - fatty streaks - atheromas
Mönckeberg's	- media calcific stenosis - "gooseneck lumps" - small and medium size arteries - asymptomatic
arteriolosclerosis (hyperplastic)	- fibrinoid necrosis - malignant hypertension - "onion skin" hyperplasia
arteriolosclerosis (hyaline)	- diabetes, hypertension, old age - thickened basement membrane

1.23.) ARTERITIS

hypersensitivity arteritis	- small vessels - lesions all at same stage - cryoglobulins - a/w Henoch Schönlein
polyarteritis nodosa	- small and medium vessels - kidney, heart, Gi tract - does not affect lung
thrombangitis obliterans (Buerger's)	- small and medium vessels - in smokers
giant cell arteritis	- temporal artery - sudden blindness - female > male ! - a/w polymyalgia rheumatica
Wegener's	- upper respiratory vasculitis - lower respiratory vasculitis - glomerulonephritis
Takayasu	- "pulseless disease" - aorta / large arteries - Asian females
Kawasaki	- mucocutaneous lymph node syndrome - fever, conjunctivitis, maculopapular rash - coronary artery aneurysms - Japanese children

1.24.) <u>ANEURYSMS</u>

atherosclerotic	- fusiform - abdominal aorta - hypertension
syphilitic	- saccular - ascending aorta - a/w aortic insufficiency
dissecting	- aorta (ascending or descending) - hypertension - Marfan's
berry	- congenital - circle of Willis - a/w polycystic kidney disease (adult form)
micro	- cerebral : hypertension - retinal : diabetes

1.25.) **HEART SOUNDS**

mitral valve prolapse	young women Marfan's	midsystolic click
mitral stenosis	atrial fibrillation	diastolic rumble
mitral regurgitation	MI (papillary muscle) rheumatic fever endocarditis	holosystolic murmur *transmitted to axilla*
aortic stenosis	congenital degenerative calcification *pulsus parvus et tardus*	systolic murmur *transmitted to carotid art.*
aortic regurgitation	"water hammer" pulse	diastolic murmur "pistol shots" in femoral art.
patent ductus arteriosus	kept open by PGE_2 , PGI_2	continuous murmur (machine like)

1.26.) <u>CONGENITAL HEART DEFECTS</u>

acyanotic (L -> R)	cyanotic (R -> L)	obstructive

- VSD[1]
- ASD
  ostium primum
  ostium secundum
 	
- PDA
	- Fallot[1]
	- transposition of great vessels
	- persistent truncus arteriosus
	- Eisenmenger : reversal
		- coarctation of aorta
		  preductal (infants)
		  postductal (adults)
		
		- pulmonary or aortic
		  stenosis or atresia

[1]most common

fetal alcohol syndrome	- microcephaly - cardiac defects - short, upturned nose, long philtrum
fetal hydantoin syndrome	- nail hypoplasia - microcephaly - cardiac defects
isotretinoin (Vit. A)	- cleft palate - hydrocephalus - cardiac defects
syphilis	- bullous skin lesions (palms, soles) - Hutchinson's teeth - saber shins
TORCH[2] (cross blood-placenta barrier)	- microcephaly - auditory and visual defects - cardiac defects

[2] **Toxoplasmosis, Rubella, CMV, Herpes**

1.27.) <u>ISCHEMIC HEART DISEASE</u>

stable angina	- exercise - ST depression - relieved by rest - *Rx : nitroglycerin*
unstable angina	- at rest, crescendo - often leads to MI - *unresponsive to nitroglycerin*
Prinzmetal's angina	- at rest - ST elevated - *Rx : Ca^{2+} antagonists*

myocardial infarction	- during exercise or REM sleep
	- ST elevation
	- T inversion
	- CK(MB) -> SGOT -> LDH1
	
	- *Rx : nitroglycerin*
	     morphine
	     lidocaine

1.28.) <u>HEART FAILURE</u>

LEFT	RIGHT
causes	
ischemic heart disease	left sided heart failure
valvular disease	lung disease[1]
hypertension	primary pulmonary hypertension
consequences	
pulmonary congestion	nutmeg liver
dyspnea, orthopnea	renal hypoperfusion
renal hypoperfusion	salt retention
salt retention	edema, ascites

 [1]*smooth muscle of pulmonary arteries contracts during hypoxia causing pulmonary hypertension!*

1.29.) <u>ENDOCARDITIS</u>

acute	subacute	marantic	Libman Sacks
- Staph. aureus - Streptococci	- Strep. viridans - gram negative bacilli	- thrombotic	- verrucous [1]
- previously normal valves	- previously abnormal valves	- a/w chronic illnesses	- SLE
- Janeway lesion	- Roth spots - Osler nodes		
- high fever, chills - hematuria	- low grade fever		

[1] *both sides of valve leaflet*

1.30.) **PERICARDITIS**

fibrinous	- myocardial infarction, - Dressler's - "bread and butter"
serous	- viral (coxsackie) - uremia
suppurative	- bacterial - fungal - parasitic

Signs :
Pericardial friction rub
Pulsus paradoxus (normal inspiratory fall in blood pressure
that is exaggerated)

1.31.) <u>RHEUMATIC DISEASES</u>

acute rheumatic fever	rheumatic heart disease
β-hemolytic streptococci	often asymptomatic
common in children	verrucae on lines of closure (mitral valve > aortic valve)

<u>major Jones criteria</u>
  - polyarthritis
  - erythema
  - subcutaneous nodules
  - chorea
  - carditis	

1.32.) <u>OBSTRUCTIVE LUNG DISEASES</u>

emphysema[1]	- **pink puffers**, barrel chest
	- **panacinar**
	  (α1-antitrypsin deficiency, lower lobes)
	- **centriacinar**
	  (smoking, upper lobes)

chronic bronchitis[1]	- **blue bloaters** - chronic irritation/ infections - hypertrophy of submucosal glands
asthma	- expiratory wheezing - extrinsic (allergic) - intrinsic (cold, exercise) - aspirin induced
bronchiectasis	- result of chronic infections - Kartagener's : immotile cilia

[1] often coexisting = COPD

1.33.) <u>RESTRICTIVE LUNG DISEASES</u>

adult ARDS	- acute diffuse alveolar damage 　(sepsis, shock, pancreatitis, toxins)
neonatal ARDS	- insufficient lecithin synthesis by type II pneumocytes
pneumoconiosis	- coal : "tattooing", black sputum - anthracosis : carbon dust - asbestosis : fibrous silicates, dry cough - berylliosis : **type IV hypersensitivity**
hypersensitivity pneumonitis	- acute : **(type III)** fever, cough, dyspnea, leukocytosis - chronic : **(type IV)** peribronchial granulomas - farmer's lung, pigeon breeder's lung etc.
Goodpasture syndrome	- **(type II)**, Ab against basal membrane - hemoptysis, rapidly progressive glomerulonephritis
pulmonary hemosiderosis	- like Goodpasture's, without renal involvement
alveolar proteinosis	- overproduction of surfactant like material
eosinophilic pneumonia	- acute (Löffler's) : **type 1** - chronic
diffuse idiopathic fibrosis	- interstitial pneumonitis and fibrosis - hyperplasia of type II pneumocytes
collagen vascular disorders	- scleroderma, SLE, Wegener's, RA etc.

1.34.) PNEUMONIA

bronchopneumonia	Hemophilus Pseudomonas
lobar pneumonia	Pneumococcus Klebsiella
atypical pneumonia [1]	viral Mycoplasma
Legionnaire's disease [2] (self-limited lobar pneumonia)	Legionnella

[1] most frequent in young adults (college students)

[2] more frequent in elderly, via water reservoirs
   no person to person transmission

1.35.) LUNG TUMORS

benign	- hamartoma - adenoma - leiomyoma etc.
carcinoid	- potentially malignant - not related to smoking - <u>carcinoid syndrome</u> suggests widespread metastasis

carcinoma	**adeno CA**
	   - peripheral, less related to smoking
	
	squamous CA
	   - central, strong correlation with smoking
	
	small cell CA
	   - central, hormone producing, aggressive
	
	large cell CA
	   - peripheral, poorly differentiated adeno or squamous CA

1.36.) <u>GLOMERULONEPHRITIS I</u>

nephritic syndrome	nephrotic syndrome
- hematuria - RBC casts	- severe proteinuria - hypoalbuminemia - hyperlipidemia - edema
- post strept. GN	- membranous GN (adults) - minimal change (children)

diffuse proliferative GN	- poststreptococcal GN - good prognosis
mesangiocapillary GN (membrano-proliferative GN)	- young adults, idiopathic - poor prognosis
focal-segmental GN	- aggressive variant of minimal change GN
Goodpasture's (anti -GBM antibodies)	- young males - pulmonary hemorrhage
Berger's (IgA nephropathy)	- same as Henoch Schönlein's - may follow resp. infection - mild proteinuria, hematuria

1.37.) GLOMERULONEPHRITIS II

			prognosis
minimal change (lipoid nephrosis)	- most common nephrotic syndrome in children - insidious onset	- no immune complexes - **loss of foot processes in EM**	good
membranous	- most common nephrotic syndrome in young adults - insidious onset	- l.m. : thickening of GBM - **subepithelial** deposits of immune complexes - 85% unknown antigen	mixed
membrano proliferative	- variable presentation	- GBM thickening plus proliferation of mesangium - **subendothelial or intra-membranous** deposits of immune complexes "tram track" appearance	very poor
focal segmental	- maybe related to minimal change - but proteinuria is nonselective	- segmental sclerosis - usually IgM deposits (**IgA in Berger's**)	poor
diffuse proliferative	- nephritic/nephrotic - post streptococcal, SLE	- proliferation of mesangium and epithelium - **subepithelial** deposits	good
rapidly progressive	- aggressive variant of other GN	- **crescents** - oliguria, uremia	very poor

1.38.) UROLITHIASIS

calcium	- 80% of all cases - precipitates in **alkaline** urine - *Rx : thiazide* *potassium phosphate*

Mg - NH₃ - Phosphate	- "triple stones"
	  (staghorn calculi)
	- following infection by Proteus
	- precipitates in **alkaline** urine
	
	- *Rx : antibiotics*
	     acidification

uric acid	- gout - leukemia - precipitates in **acidic** urine - *Rx : bicarbonate*
cystine	- congenital defect in dibasic amino acid transporter - precipitates in **acidic** urine - *Rx : bicarbonate*

1.39.) <u>VENEREAL DISEASES</u>

Disease	Organism	Presentation	Treatment
condyloma acuminatum	HPV	"red warts"	Rx : cryotherapy
syphilis (I) syphilis (II) syphilis (III)	Treponema pallidum	hard chancre (painless) cond. lata (flat brown papules) gumma	Rx : penicillin G
chancroid	Hemophilus ducreii	soft chancre (painful)	Rx : ceftriaxone
lymphogranuloma venerum	Chlamydia trachomatis	ulcer (painless) lymphadenopathy	Rx : doxycycline
granuloma inguinale	C. donovani	multiple ulcerating papules lymph nodes not involved [1]	Rx : tetracycline
trichomoniasis	Trichomonas vaginalis	men : asymptomatic or NGU female : vaginitis	Rx : metronidazole
genital herpes	HSV2 or HSV1	recurrent vesicles (painful)	Rx : acyclovir
candidiasis [2]	Candida albicans	female : vaginitis	Rx : nystatin, niconazole

[1] induration is of subcutaneous tissue   [2] listed here for comparison, but candidiasis is not considered to be a VD !!!

35

1.40.) TESTES TUMORS

Germ Cell Tumors (most common)

seminoma	- uniform polyhedral - radiosensitive
embryonal	- more aggressive - hemorrhage, necrosis
choriocarcinoma	- highly malignant - gynecomastia - HCG
yolk sac	- most common in children - AFP, α1-antitrypsin - very aggressive
teratoma	- childhood - fairly benign

Non Germ Cell Tumors (rare)

Leydig cell	- androgens, estrogens corticosteroids
Sertoli cell	- little hormone production
lymphoma	- most common in elderly

Tumor markers : AFP : all germ cell CA except choriocarcinoma
HCG : all germ cell CA except yolk sac carcinoma

1.41.) OVARIAN TUMORS

Surface Endothelium (most common)

serous	cysts, ciliated epithelium
mucinous	cysts, non ciliated epithelium
endometroid	glandular
clear cell	rare, malignant
Brenner	rare, benign nests of transitional epithelium in stroma

Germ Cell Tumors

teratoma	mature (dermoid cyst) or immature
dysgerminoma	= seminoma, radiosensitive
endodermal sinus tumor	= yolk sac tumor, AFP, α1-antitrypsin
choriocarcinoma	HCG

Stroma Cell Tumors

granulosa-theca	estrogens and androgens
Sertoli-Leydig	androgens
fibroma	Meig's syndrome

1.42.) <u>ENDOMETRIUM</u>

polyps	hyperplasia	carcinoma
- excessive bleeding - rarely malignant transformation	- excessive bleeding - premalignant	- usually adeno CA - may be asymptomatic or unusual discharge - <u>**risk factors**</u> estrogens obesity, diabetes hypertension infertility

1.43.) <u>PLACENTA</u>

hydatidiform mole	choriocarcinoma
- older pregnant woman - uterus larger than expected - grape-like cystic material - 80% benign - HCG elevated	- derived from : hydatidiform mole (50%) pregnancy (25%) abortion (25%) - HCG elevated - frequent metastases

1.44.) BREAST

fibrocystic disease	breast cancer
- often bilateral - multiple nodules - menstrual variation - may regress during pregnancy	- often unilateral - single mass - no cyclic variations

BENIGN TUMORS

fibroadenoma	- single, movable nodule
cystosarcoma phyllodes	- rapidly growing
intraductal papilloma	- nipple discharge (bloody or serous) - nipple retraction

MALIGNANT TUMORS

ductal carcinoma	- (most common)
lobular carcinoma	- (often receptor positive)
Paget's	- older woman - nipple involved - poor prognosis

 Risk factors for breast cancer:
nulliparity, early menarche
late menopause, fibrocystic disease

1.45.) <u>MOUTH</u>

bleeding gums	Vit. C deficiency
glossitis, cheilosis	Vit. B2 deficiency
smooth beefy red tongue	Vit. B12 deficiency
strawberry tongue	scarlet fever
Koplik's spots (white dots on red background)	measles
thrush (white, removable)	Candida albicans

1.46.) <u>ESOPHAGEAL DIVERTICULAS</u>

Pulsion Diverticula (Zenker's)	Traction Diverticula
- "false" (mucosa only)	- "true" (all layers)
- at junction of pharynx/esophagus	- midpart of esophagus
- dysphagia, regurgitation	- asymptomatic

1.47.) GASTRITIS

acute	chronic A	chronic B	Ménétrier's
- alcohol - NSAIDs - stress	- fundal gastritis - autoimmune - pernicious anemia	- antral gastritis - H. pylori	- thickened mucosa

1.48.) GASTROENTERITIS

toxin ingestion	bacteria	non-bacterial
Staph. aureus Cl. botulinum	toxigenic Campylobacter E.coli Salmonella invasive Shigella	Rotavirus (children) Parvovirus (adults) Candida Entameba histolytica Giardia lamblia

1.49.) <u>POLYPOSIS OF COLON</u>

familial multiple polyposis	auto-dominant	- polyps only	cancer risk 100%
Peutz-Jegher's	auto-dominant	- polyps plus : - melanin pigmentation of lips, palms, soles	no cancer risk
Gardner's	auto-dominant	- polyps plus : - tumor of skin and bones	cancer risk 100%
Turcot's	auto-recessive	- polyps plus : - brain tumors	low cancer risk

1.50.) __INFLAMMATORY BOWEL DISEASE__

Crohn's	Ulcerative colitis
rectum often spared **ileum often involved**	**begins at rectum and progresses** **towards ileocecal junction**
skip lesions transmural	continuous mucosa / submucosa only
granulomas strictures and fissures	crypt abscesses pseudopolyps
more pain, less bleeding	more bleeding, less pain
	increased risk for colon cancer

1.51.) __MALABSORPTION__

celiac sprue	- toxic/allergic reaction against gluten - avoid wheat - rice and corn o.k.
tropical sprue	- E.coli enterotoxin ?
Whipple's	- systemic disease - a/w arthritis - gram ⊢ bacilli found in lamina propria - *Rx : penicillin or tetracycline*

1.52.) CHOLELITHIASIS

cholesterol	mixed	pigment
- radiolucent - Westerners - **fat, female, forty, fertile**	- 15% radiopaque	- radiolucent - Asians

Porcelain Gallbladder : - calcium deposits in wall
- high risk of malignancy

Strawberry Gallbladder : - asymptomatic lipid deposits
- not related to cholelithiasis
- no cancer risk

1.53.) CARCINOMA

gallbladder CA	bile duct CA
- female - cholelithiasis - porcelain gallbladder	- male - chronic infections - liver fluke (Clonorchis sinensis)

1.54.) JAUNDICE

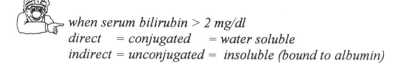

when serum bilirubin > 2 mg/dl
direct   = conjugated   = water soluble
indirect = unconjugated = insoluble (bound to albumin)

prehepatic	hemolysis
hepatic	hepatitis
posthepatic	cholestasis

Congenital causes of jaundice :

Gilbert	auto-dominant	impaired conjugation (mild)
Crigler-Najar	auto-dominant or auto-recessive	impaired conjugation (very severe)
Rotor	auto-recessive	impaired hepatocellular secretion

1.55.) HEPATITIS

A	RNA	- viruses in feces - acute : IgM - late : IgG	- **fecal/oral** - 2-6 weeks [2] - 0% chronic
B	DNA	- HBs-Ag , earliest marker[1] - HBe-Ag, infective state	- **parenteral** - 2-6 months [2] - 10% chronic
C	RNA	- antibody ELISA	- **parenteral** - 1-2 months [2] - 50% chronic
Delta	RNA	- requires HBV's Ag coat (superinfection)	- **parenteral**
E	RNA		- **fecal oral** - SE Asia - fulminant in pregnant woman

[1] also indicates carrier state   [2] incubation times

1.56.) TOXIC HEPATITIS

predictable	**idiosyncratic**
amanita acetaminophen carbon tetrachloride methotrexates	halothane isoniazid methyl-DOPA

1.57.) CIRRHOSIS

alcohol	postnecrotic	biliary
60%	30%	10%
early : micronodular late : macronodular	macronodular	micronodular
Mallory bodies in acute hepatitis !		auto-immune disease anti-mitochondrial antibodies

1.58.) LIVER CARCINOMA

metastatic	hepatocellular	cholangiocarcinoma
most common	90% of all primary ones	10% of primary ones

from breast
from lung
from colon
	does not metastasize
	
	AFP marker
		metastasizes to:
		    lungs
		    bones
		    brain

1.59.) <u>ARTHRITIS</u>

Osteoarthritis	Rheumatoid Arthritis (RA)
- loss of cartilage - narrowing of joint space	- erosions, osteoporosis
- vertebrae, hips, knees - distal interphalangeal joints - joint stiffness - Heberden's nodes	- starts in small joints - malaise, morning stiffness - rheumatoid nodules (skin, valves etc.)

Still's disease :
juvenile RA, acute febrile, no rheumatoid factors

Psoriatic arthritis:
like RA, but absence of rheumatoid factors

Felty's disease :
polyarticular RA, splenomegaly, leukopenia, leg ulcers

1.60.) BONES

osteogenesis imperfecta	- disorder of collagen synthesis - fractures - blue, thin sclera
osteopetrosis	- increased density - brittle bones
achondroplasia	- defective cartilage synthesis - decreased epiphyseal formation
aseptic necrosis	- head of femur - navicular bone

osteoporosis	osteomalacia	Paget's

- thinned cortical bone
- enlarged medullary cavity
 	
- normal Ca and phosphate
- normal alk. phosphatase
	- diffuse radiolucency
	
	- low Ca, low phosphate
	- high alk. phosphatase
		- bones enlarged and
		  radiolucent
		
		- extremely high alk.
		  phosphatase

- decrease in bone mass
- estrogen deficiency
- immobilization
- Cushing's
	- impaired mineralization
	- lack of Vit. D
	- chronic renal
	  insufficiency
		- excessive bone resorption
		  with replacement.

1.61.) <u>CARTILAGE TUMORS</u>

osteochondroma	- developmental defect - exostosis at metaphyseal projections
enchondroma	- may develop into chondrosarcoma - cartilage within bone
chondroblastoma	- benign - femur, tibia, humerus epiphysis
chondrosarcoma	- malignant - spine, pelvic bones - slower growing than osteosarcoma

1.62.) <u>BONE TUMORS</u>

osteoma	- benign - skull
osteoid osteoma	- benign, painful - tibia or femur (diaphysis)
osteoblastoma	- like osteoid osteoma - larger but painless - may be malignant
osteosarcoma	- highly malignant - metaphysis of long bone (knee) - Codman's triangle
Ewing's sarcoma	- young males - pelvis, long bones - within marrow cavity - "onion skin" appearance - very aggressive

1.63.) <u>MUSCULAR DYSTROPHIES</u>

Duchenne	- X linked - most severe - pelvic girdle weakness - pseudohypertrophy (lower limbs)
Becker	- X linked - less severe than Duchenne - may walk until age 20-25
limb girdle	- auto recessive - **late** onset
facioscapulohumeral	- auto dominant - **late** onset
myotonic	- auto dominant - **late** onset - limb involvement is distal - inability to voluntarily relax muscle

1.64.) BRAIN TUMORS

Neural Tube (gliomas)	astrocytoma	- slow growing, M > F
	glioblastoma	- always fatal, M > F
	medulloblastoma	- children, M > F CSF cytology !
	oligodendroblastoma	- rare, M = F slow growing, seizures
Neural Crest	meningioma	- from arachnoid, benign, F > M "whorling pattern", psammoma bodies
	Schwannoma	- acoustic neurinoma, F > M a/w von Recklinghausen's
	neurofibroma	- fibroblasts and Schwann cells, benign usually von Recklinghausen's
ctoderm	craniopharyngioma	- most common supratentorial tumor in children, compresses optic nerve
	pituitary adenoma	- 60% prolactin (chromophobe) - 10% growth hormone (eosinophil) - 10% ACTH (basophil)
esoderm	lymphoma	- B cells, periventricular
	lipoma	- "egg shell" appearance
	hemangioblastoma	

1.65.) CNS DEGENERATION

Alzheimer's	- most common - diffuse cortical atrophy
Pick's	- lobar atrophy - mainly frontal and temporal
Parkinson's	- bradykinesia, rigidity, resting tremor - dopamine depletion (caudate, putamen) - Lewy bodies
Friedreich's ataxia	- autosomal recessive - pes cavus - loss of proprioception - tremors, Babinsky - spinal cord atrophy (spinocerebellar, corticospinal, post. columns)

1.66.) TIA

internal carotid artery	vertebrobasilar artery
- monocular blindness, ipsilateral *"amaurosis fugax"* - hemiparesis, contralateral - hemisensory loss, contralateral - language disturbance	- vertigo - diplopia - ataxia - facial numbness/weakness - nausea

1.67.) <u>DEMYELINATION</u>

multiple sclerosis	- onset at age 20-40 - a/w cool, temperate climate - IgG (oligoclonal bands) in CSF
Devic's	- like M.S., but limited to spinal chord and optical nerve
Guillain-Barré	- peripheral nerves (mainly motor) - autoimmune, often following viral infection
adrenoleukodystrophy	- X linked - accumulation of long chain cholesterols - blindness, ataxia - latent adrenal insufficiency
Schilder's	- focal demyelination in brain - children - visual, auditory, motor defects - variant of adrenoleukodystrophy

1.68.) PITUITARY HYPERFUNCTION

eosinophile	prolactin	male : decreased libido, impotence female : galactorrhea, amenorrhea, infertility
	GH	prepubertal : giantism adults : acromegaly
basophile	ACTH	Cushing's disease (most common cause of Cushing's syndrome except iatrogenic)

Classification according to staining properties is outdated since there is only an approximate relationship between hormones and cell staining.

 While prolactin is mainly produced by eosinophil cells, prolactinomas are usually chromophobe !

1.69.) PITUITARY HYPOFUNCTION

Sheehan's (ischemic necrosis, postpartum)	panhypopituitarism - hypothyroidism - hypoadrenalism - hypogonadism
dwarfism	a) growth hormone deficiency b) lack of receptors (eg. in pygmies)
eunuchoid hypogonadism, primary amenorrhea	gonadotropin deficiency (common !)

1.70.) ADRENAL ADENOMAS/CARCINOMAS

Cortex : Adenoma	most nonfunctional, i.e. do not produce steroids
Cortex : Carcinoma	most produce steroids - Conn : mineralcorticoids - Cushing : glucocorticoids - virilization : androgens
Medulla : Pheochromocytoma	10% extra-adrenal 10% bilateral 10% malignant
Medulla : Neuroblastoma	malignant medulla or sympathetic chain ganglia

Mineral corticoids	zona **g**lomerulosa
Glucocorticoids	zona **f**asciculata
Androgens	zona **r**eticularis

 "the deeper you go the sweeter it gets"

1.71.) <u>THYROID</u>

Hyperthyroidism :	**Graves'** (diffuse toxic goiter)	- lymphocytes - small follicles - little colloid
	Plummer's (nodular toxic goiter)	- hyperplasia, hypertrophy - colloid accumulation
Hypothyroidism :	**diffuse simple goiter** (iodine deficiency)	- hyperplasia, hypertrophy
	Hashimoto's	- lymphocytes, plasma cells - atrophic follicles - little colloid
	Riedel's	- fibrous replacement
Euthyroid :	**De Quervain's**	- viral - leakage of colloid - granulomas

1.72.) <u>THYROID-TUMORS</u>

benign :	follicular adenoma	-very common - most are cold nodules
malignant :	papillary CA	- most common malignant - Psammoma bodies
	follicular CA	- adenomatous pattern - more malignant than papillary CA
	anaplastic CA	- undifferentiated - poor prognosis
	medullary CA	- parafollicular (C cells)

1.73.) <u>PARATHYROIDS</u>

Hyperparathyroidism	primary	- adenoma (most common)
	secondary	- chronic renal failure - Vit.D deficiency
Hypoparathyroidism		- thyroidectomy, radiation - DiGeorge's syndrome **- PTH low** **- Ca^{2+} low**
Pseudohypo...		- Albright's - short stature, round face - receptor defect **- PTH elevated** **- Ca^{2+} low**
Pseudopseudohypo...		- same physical appearance as in pseudohypoparathyroidism **- PTH normal** **- Ca^{2+} levels normal**

1.74.) <u>DIABETES</u>

IDDM	NIDDM	MODY
- juvenile - prone to ketoacidosis - viral - genetic - auto-immune (islet cell antibodies)	- adult - not prone to ketoacidosis - inadequate insulin secretion - insulin resistance	- juvenile onset - like NIDDM - glucokinase defect (glucose sensor)

1.75.) <u>MULTIPLE ENDOCRINE NEOPLASMS</u>

MEN I	MEN IIa	MEN IIb
adrenal <u>cortex</u> pituitary parathyroid pancreas (gastrinoma)	adrenal <u>medulla</u> thyroid medulla parathyroid	adrenal <u>medulla</u> thyroid medulla neurofibroma
"pity-para-pan"	"para-medullary-medulla"	

1.76.) <u>TOXICOLOGY</u>

cadmium	"honeycomb" pneumonitis
cobalt	cardiomyopathy
lead	inhibits heme synthesis renal tubular acidosis
mercury	neurotoxic (Minamata !) proximal tubular necrosis
arsenic	lung cancer
asbestos	mesothelioma
aromatic amines	bladder cancer
benzene	leukemia
chromium	lung cancer
vinyl chloride	liver angiosarcoma
CO	forms carboxyhemoglobin[1]
α-amanitin	fulminant hepatitis

[1] do not confuse with methemoglobin, which contains oxidized Fe^{3+}

1.77.) DERMATOLOGY

seborrhoic keratosis	brownish/gray, scaly, greasy
keratocanthoma	rapidly growing pink papula looks like squamous cell carcinoma but is benign
actinic keratosis	crusty red papule, premalignant
basal cell carcinoma	pearly, gray papule
squamous cell carcinoma	erythematous, scaly or oozing ulcer Bowen's disease: squamous CA in situ
xanthoma	hyperlipidemia, foamy histocytes

capillary hemangioma	- "salmon patches" and stork bites
	   spontaneously regress
	- "strawberry hemangiomas"
	   initially grow, later regress

cavernous hemangioma	- portwine stain, a/w Sturge-Weber *do not resolve spontaneously*
cafe au lait spots	a/w von Recklinghausen's
vitiligo	irregular depigmentation
melanoma	brown, black, red, white, purple, irregular borders lentigo maligna : grows horizontally nodular melanoma : grows vertically

1.78.) <u>MORE DERMATOLOGY</u>

pemphigus	vesicles on mucosa auto antibodies against intercellular junctions of keratinocytes
pemphigoid	like pemphigus, but larger bullae on abdomen, groin ...
impetigo	honey colored crust, superficial skin infection β hemolytic strep. or staph
pityriasis	(viral ?), herald patch -> spreads along flexural lines
rosacea	large, red nose

MICROBIOLOGY

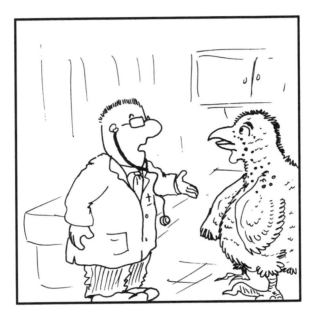

"It could be chicken pox, but then all these
viruses look similar."

2.1.) <u>STAINING</u>

Ziehl Neelson	acid fast bacteria
Giemsa	blood cells
PAS	glycogen, mucopolysaccharides
congo red	amyloid
osmic acid	electron microscopy

2.2.) <u>NORMAL FLORA</u>

skin	Staph. epidermidis
nose	Staph. aureus
mouth	Strep. viridans
colon	Bacteroides fragilis
vagina	Lactobacillus

2.3.) <u>CELL WALLS</u>

all (except mycobacteria)	- peptidoglycans - D-alanine - diaminopimelic acid
gram positive	- teichoic acid
gram negative	- lipopolysaccharide (endotoxin) - outer cell membrane, porins
mycobacteria	- mycolic acid
mycoplasma	- no cell wall - have sterols
spores	- dipicolinic acid

2.4.) <u>TOXINS</u>

ENDOTOXINS	- lipopolysaccharide - non-specific - TNF, IL-1 --> fever, shock - poor antigen - heat stabile
EXOTOXINS	- polypeptide - specific - toxoids used as vaccine - usually heat labile
- tetanus toxin	- blocks release of glycin
- botulinum toxin	- blocks release of ACh
- diphtheria toxin	- inhibits protein synthesis - (ADP-ribosylation of EF-2)
- alpha toxin	- lecithinase (gas gangrene)
- toxic shock syndr. toxin	- Staph. aureus - induces IL-1, IL-2 - identical with enterotoxin F
- cholera toxin	- stimulates adenylate cyclase (activates G_s)
- pertussis toxin	- stimulates adenylate cyclase (inhibits G_i)
- enterotoxin (E.coli)	- heat labile: stim. adenylate cyclase - heat stabile: stim. guanylate cyclase

2.5.) <u>O_2-REQUIREMENTS</u>

obligate aerobe	tubercle bacillus B. anthracis Nocardia
micro aerophilic	Brucella abortus Campylobacter jejuni
obligate anaerobe	Clostridium Actinomyces
facultative anaerobe	most others

2.6.) STAPHYLOCOCCI
(Catalase +)

	coagulase	novobiocin	
S. aureus	+		skin infections osteomyelitis endocarditis toxic shock syndrome food poisoning
S. epidermidis	-	sensitive	infections following: instrumentation implants etc.
S. saprophyticus	-	insensitive	UTI

Exotoxins:
Enterotoxin A-F
Toxic shock syndrome toxin
Exfoliatin (scalded skin)
Alpha toxin (tissue necrosis)

2.7.) <u>STREPTOCOCCI</u>
(Catalase -)

ß-hemolytic	**- complete hemolysis (clear halo)**
	
	- <u>Strept. pyogenes</u> (Group A)[1]
	    bacitracin sensitive
	- <u>other Strept</u>. (Groups B-T)[1]
	    bacitracin insensitive

α-hemolytic	**- incomplete hemolysis (green halo)**
	- <u>Pneumococci</u>
	    bile soluble (lysis)
	    optochin sensitive
	- <u>Strept. viridans</u>
	    bile insoluble
	    optochin insensitive

γ-hemolytic	**- no hemolysis** - Enterococci (Group D)[1]

[1] C-antigen, <u>c</u>ell-wall, determines group (=Lancefield antigen)

compared to staphylococci :   - grow better on enriched medium
                                     - narrower temperature range
                                     - in culture : small colonies, no pigment

Exotoxins:
Streptokinase
Streptodornase (DNAse)
Hyaluronidase
Erythrogenic toxin
Streptolysin O
Streptolysin S

2.8.)   <u>NEISSERIA</u>
(gram - oxidase +)

Meningococcus	- has capsule - ferments maltose - Waterhouse-Friderichson - *Rx : penicillin G*

Gonococcus	- has pilus
	- does not ferment maltose
	
	- male : dysuria, purulent discharge
	- female: endocervix infections
	                salpingitis
	                infertility
	- both: septic arthritis (common !)
	
	- *Rx : ceftriaxone*
	          tetracycline[1]

 [1] *coexisting C.trachomatis infection is very common.*

2.9.) <u>BACILLI</u>

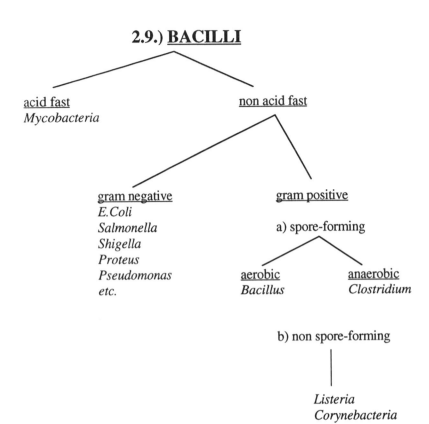

<u>acid fast</u>
Mycobacteria

<u>non acid fast</u>

<u>gram negative</u>
E.Coli
Salmonella
Shigella
Proteus
Pseudomonas
etc.

<u>gram positive</u>

a) spore-forming

<u>aerobic</u>
Bacillus

<u>anaerobic</u>
Clostridium

b) non spore-forming

Listeria
Corynebacteria

2.10.) <u>GRAM + BACILLI</u>

	aerobe	toxins	spores	
Bacillus	+	+	+	- anthrax - woolsorter's disease - "fried rice" poisoning

Coryne b.	+	+	-	- diphtheria
				    pseudomembranes
				    Loeffler's telluride
				    "Chinese characters"

Listeria	+	-	-	- sepsis, meningitis - neonates or immunosuppressed - "Chinese characters" + motile !
Clostridium	-	+	+	- tetanus - botulism - gas gangrene (α-toxin) - food poisoning (reheated meat) - pseudomembranous colitis
Lactobacillus	-	-	-	- prefers acidic pH - protects GI and vagina

2.11.) <u>CLOSTRIDIA</u>

Cl. botulinum	- non-capsulate, sporing, motile - types A-G (antigenically different exotoxins)
Cl. tetani	- non-capsulate, sporing, motile - 10 types (flagellar antigen) - but all have the same exotoxin

Cl. perfringens	- non-capsulate, sporing, non-motile
	- α toxin = lecithinase
	  causes gas gangrene in soldiers
	- enterotoxin (heat labile)
	  causes food poisoning (reheated meat stews)

2.12.) ENTEROBACTERIACEAE
(fac. anaerobe, glucose + oxidase -)

Gram negative bacilli. 5 major genera. All look the same, some are motile, some are not. Differentiated by cultural appearance and biochemical activities. Subtyping is done by serology.

E. coli	- motile - lactose + - indole -
Salmonella	- motile - lactose - - indole - - S.typhi produces gas, 1500 other salmonellas don't a) food poisoning : inc. 1-2 days b) enteric fever (typhoid, paratyphoid), inc. 10-14 days
Shigella	- non-motile - lactose - - indole +, but no gas - **dysentriae** (serious), **flexneri, boydii, sonnei** (mild)
Proteus	- motile (swarm !) - produce urease --> ammonium calculi with UTI - have antigens that crossreact with anti-rickettsia ABs (Weil-Felix reaction) - do not cause gastroenteritis
Klebsiella	- non-motile - lactose + - produce lots of slime (M antigen) - pneumonia ("currant jelly" sputum)

K-antigen: Capsule,   H-antigen: Flagella,   O-antigen: surface

2.13.) <u>ENTEROBACTERIACEAE - DX</u>

	Shigella	Salmonella	E. Coli
motile	no	yes	yes
gas from glucose	no	yes[1]	yes
H₂S production	no	yes	yes
ferments lactose	no	no	yes

[1]only S.typhi !

 Shigella is 1000x more infective than Salmonella.

2.14.) <u>MORE ENTEROBACTERIACEAE</u>

Bacteroides fragilis	- most common cause of gram - infections ! - anaerobic, likes bile - forms abscess - *Rx : metronidazole*
Vibrio cholera	- comma shaped - rice-watery diarrhea (non bloody) - *Rx : tetracycline*
Vibrio parahemolyticus	- diarrhea in Japan (sushi-lovers) - "salt resistant" - *self-limited*
Campylobacter jejuni	- very common in US - grows best at 5% CO_2, 42°C - watery, foul smelling stools later may be bloody - *Rx : erythromycin, aminoglycoside*
Helicobacter pylori	- very similar to Campylobacter (but urease +) - damages gastric mucosa - *Rx : amoxicillin, metronidazole*

2.15.) GRAM - BACILLI (ZOONOTIC)

Yersinia pestis
"black death"
	- bubonic plague
	   rodents -> fleas -> humans
	   large, very tender lymph nodes
	
	- pulmonary plague
	   humans -> humans
	
	- *Rx : streptomycin, tetracycline*

Pasteurella	- bipolar staining - wound infections (dog and cat bites) - cellulitis, osteomyelitis - *Rx : penicillin G*
Brucella	- undulating fever - Br. abortus (placentitis in cows) - Br. melitensis (goats and sheep) - Br. suis (pigs) - *Rx : tetracycline, gentamycin*
Francisella	- tularemia - rabbits -> ticks -> humans - influenza like, adenopathy - *Rx : streptomycin*

2.16.) <u>GRAM - BACILLI (OTHER)</u>

Pseudomonas	- does not ferment glucose - oxidase + - musty odor, greenish bluish pigment (pus) - common wound infection (burns) - pneumonia, UTI - *resists most antibiotics and disinfectants*
Hemophilus	- requires blood (chocolate agar) - requires factor V and X. - grows around staphylococci (satellites) - H. influenza : bronchitis, meningitis - H. ducreyii : chancroid - H. hemolyticus : may be confused with S. pyogenes (but is gram - and resists bacitracin)
Bordetella	- looks like Hemophilus - pertussis toxin (whooping cough) - requires Bordet-Gengou, not chocolate agar - *Rx : erythromycin*
Legionella	- gram - cell wall, but stains only faintly - atypical pneumonia - grows in water reservoirs - no cold agglutinins ! - *Rx : erythromycin*

2.17.) MYCOBACTERIA

M. tuberculosis	- slow respiratory infection - primary lesion: Ghon complex - most disease due to reactivation
M. bovis	- unpasteurized milk - GI tuberculosis

M. leprae	- prefers 32°C (rather than 37°C)
	- found in nasal secretions and skin lesions
	- tuberculoid leprosy: granulomas
	                       skin test positive
	- lepromatous leprosy: nodular skin lesions
	                       skin test negative

Atypical

M. marinum	- swimming pool granuloma
M. avium-intracellulare	- clinically indistinguishable from TBC - highly resistant to therapy
M. fortuitum	- saprophyte - rapidly growing - highly resistant to therapy

2.18.) <u>HIGHER BACTERIA</u>

Actinomyces	Nocardia
- "lump jaw"	- "madura foot"
- normal mouth flora - gram positive, (acid fast) - anaerobe	- soil - (gram positive), acid fast - obligate aerobe

- *Rx : penicillin G*
    surgical drainage
	- *Rx : trimethoprim- sulfamethoxazole*
	    surgical drainage

2.19.) <u>SPIROCHETES</u>

T. pallidum	- Syphilis - related diseases: Yaws, Bejel, Pinta - *Rx : penicillin G*
B. burgdorferi	- Lyme disease - tick bite (mainly east coast) - *Rx : acute: tetracycline* *chronic: penicillin G*
B. recurrentis	- relapsing fever - antigens undergo variations (relapses) - human -> louse -> human - *Rx : tetracycline*
L. interrogans	- leptospirosis - sewers, water contaminated with rat urine - fever, jaundice, hemorrhage, uremia - *Rx : penicillin G*

2.20.) <u>CHLAMYDIA</u>

C. trachomatis	**different strains cause different diseases :**
	- urethritis (most common non-GO urethritis !)
	- lymphogranuloma venerum (purulent, but often asymptomatic in male)
	- trachoma chronic conjunctivitis that leads to blindness
	- Rx : tetracycline
C. psittaci	**- pneumonia**, sometimes with hepatitis - found in bird feces
	- Rx : tetracycline

 Giemsa stain shows cytoplasmic inclusions.

 <u>Life cycle of chlamydiae</u>:
Elementary body ->
enter cells ->
reticulate body ->
multiplication ->
release of many new elementary bodies

2.21.) <u>RICKETTSIA</u>

		vector	reservoir
Typhus: epidemic	R. prowazekii	lice	humans
endemic	R. typhi	fleas	rodents
scrub	R. tsutsugamushi	mite	rodents
Spotted fever	R. rickettsiae	ticks	dogs, rodents
Q fever	C. burnetii	-	cattle, sheep
Trench fever	R. quintana	lice	humans

- **Weil-Felix reaction** : anti-rickettsial antibodies in patient's serum crossreact with proteus antigens

- *Rx : tetracycline*

88

2.22.) <u>DNA VIRUSES</u>

- **all double stranded genome except parvovirus**
- **all icosahedral except poxvirus**

Parvo	B19	- erythema infectiosum, **5th disease** "slapped cheek"
Papova	Papilloma	- skin warts, genital warts - multiply in squamous cells
	JC	- leukoencephalopathy in immunocompromised patients
Adeno	(non-enveloped)	- respiratory infections - atypical pneumonia - conjunctivitis - gastroenteritis - hemorrhagic cystitis
Pox	Variola	- small pox
	Vaccinia	- cowpox (recombinant ?)
	Molluscum contagiosum	- small, pink warts
Hepadna	HBV	- serum hepatitis B - liver cell carcinoma

2.23.) <u>HERPES VIRUSES</u>

(ds DNA)

	Disease	Latency Phase
HSV1 **HSV2**	- mainly oral - mainly genital - both multiply in fibroblasts	trigeminal ganglion sacral DRG
VZV	- varicella, shingles	thoracolumbar DRG
EBV	- infectious mononucleosis - a/w Burkitt's lymphoma (Africa) - a/w nasopharyngioma (China)	B lymphocytes
CMV	- cytomegalic inclusion disease - heterophil negative mononucleosis (no pharyngitis !)	leukocytes
HHV-6	- roseola, **6th disease**	T lymphocytes
HHV-7	- unknown	unknown

2.24.) <u>RNA VIRUSES</u>

Picorna	Hepatitis A	- infectious hepatitis
	Polio	- paralysis (α-motoneuron)
	Coxsackie A	- herpangina
		- hand/foot/mouth disease
	Coxsackie B	- myocarditis
		- Bornholm's disease
		- A and B: meningitis
	Echo	- meningitis, URI, diarrhea
	Rhino	- common cold
Reo	Rota	- gastroenteritis (children)
Orthomyxo	Influenza A, B, C	- subtle drifts
		- major shifts
Paramyxo	**Rubeola**	**- measles**
		- encephalitis
		- SSPE
	Mumps	- parotitis, orchitis
	RSV	- bronchiolitis, pneumonia
	Parainfluenza	- croup (subglottitis)
Toga	**Rubella**	**- German measles**
	Arbo	- encephalitis
		(arthropod vectors)

2.25.) __ARBO VIRUSES__
(arthropod borne)

GENUS	MEMBER		
Toga	Alpha virus	- EEE - WEE	mosquito
Flavi	Flavi virus	- St. Louis encephalitis - yellow fever - Dengue	mosquito
Bunya	Bunya virus Hanta virus	- California encephalitis - fulminant respiratory inf.	mosquito deer mice[1]
Reo	Orbi virus	Colorado tick fever	tick

[1] *this one is an exception : no arthropod vector! No human to human transmission!*

2.26.) <u>SLOW VIRUSES</u>

AIDS	HIV
subacute sclerosing panencephalitis	measles virus
progressive multifocal leukoencephalopathy	JC virus
kuru	?
Creutzfeld-Jakob	prions
scrapie	prions
bovine spongiform encephalopathy	?

2.27.) <u>HIV</u>

genome	- ss +polarity RNA - two identical strands
gag	- internal core protein: p24 (serologic marker)
pol	- reverse transcriptase - integrase - protease
env	- gp41, gp120 (glycoproteins in lipid envelope) - **gp41 : mediates cell fusion** - **gp120 : binds to CD4 receptor** (mutates rapidly !)
tat	- regulatory gene - "transactivation of transcription" - also suppresses synthesis of class I MHC proteins

- *ELISA :*   *very sensitive*
                not very specific

- *Western blot :*   *very specific*
                      is done to confirm a positive ELISA

2.28.) <u>FUNGI</u>

A)   HOW THEY REPRODUCE

Most fungi are both, sexual and asexual.
Sexual means : 2 cells fuse, diploid cell divides by meiosis.
Asexual means : haploid cell divides by mitosis.

Fungi that do not reproduce sexually are called *fungi imperfecti*
(or maybe they have sex so rarely, that their spores went undetected so far)

Sexual spores : Ascospores, Basidiospores and Zygospores
Asexual spores are called conidia :   Arthroconidia
                                            Chlamydioconidia
                                            many more...

B)   WHAT THEY LOOK LIKE

Most are dimorphic : **yeasts** at 37°C, **molds** outside the human body.

yeasts	dimorphic fungi	molds
- **candida** thrush, vaginitis - **cryptococcus** pneumonia, meningitis	- **histoplasma** disseminated - **blastomyces** resp. tract - **coccidioides** desert rheumatism	- **aspergillos** farmer's lung - **mucor** tissue necrosis, of nose and lungs

	yeasts	molds
asexual	Blastoconidia (="buds") Pseudohyphae	Arthroconidia Chlamydioconidia etc.
sexual	Ascospores	Basidiospores Zygospores

2.29.) FUNGAL DISEASES

cutaneous	- **dermatophytosis** [1] (ringworm) - **tinea versicolor**	- hyphae - hyphae
subcutaneous	- **mycetoma** - **sporotrichosis**	- "tree" shaped (sporangia) - cigar shaped budding yeast

systemic	- **coccidioidomycosis**
	
	- **histoplasmosis**
	- **blastomycosis**
		- soil: arthrospores
		  tissue: endospores
		- yeasts in macrophages
		- broad based bud with
		  double refractory walls

opportunistic	- **cryptococcosis** - **candidiasis** - **aspergillosis**	- capsule on India ink prep. - pseudohyphae germ tubes - V shaped

[1] microsporum, trichophyton and epidermophyton

 Diagnosis by light microscopy : 10% KOH prep
(dissolves tissue but not fungal wall)

2.30.) <u>MALARIA</u>

Mosquito : **sexual cycle ->**   forms sporozoites
Human :   **asexual cycle ->**   forms schizonts

1.)   **Sporozoites** are introduced into blood
2.)   Exo-erythrocytic phase: sporozoites differentiate into merozoites
3.)   **Merozoites** settle in liver (latent forms called hypnozoites)
4.)   Liver releases merozoites
5.)   Merozoites infect red blood cells
6.)   Ringshaped **trophozoite** matures, forms multinucleated schizonts
7.)   RBC releases either 10-20 new merozoites **or gametocytes**

Vivax	- 48 h - latent liver forms
Ovale	- 48 h - latent liver forms
Falciparum	- 48 h - most severe, life threatening - no trophozoites/schizonts found in blood - banana shaped gametozytes
Malariae	- 72 h

2.31.) <u>TISSUE PROTOZOA</u>

Pneumocystis carinii	- probably a fungus,
	  however antifungal drugs are ineffective !
	- sudden onset fever, dyspnea, tachypnea
	
	*- Rx : trimethoprim-sulfamethoxazole
	     pentamidine*

Toxoplasma gondii	- cat feces, undercooked meat (pork)
	- ingestion: cysts
	- invade gut wall
	- differentiate into trophozoites (tachyzoites)
	- tachyzoites may invade brain, muscle and
	  form slowly growing cysts (bradyzoites)
	
	*- Rx : sulfonamide (first trimester)
	     sulfonamide-pyrimethamine (all others)*

Leishmania
 	
- L. donovani
 	
- L. brasiliensis
- L. mexicana
- L. tropica
	
	- Kala-Azar (**visceral**)
	  "black sickness"
	- Espundia (**mucocutaneous**)
	- **cutaneous** leishmaniosis
	  (red papule, satellites, ulcerating)
	
	- Rx : sodium stibogluconate

Trypanosoma - T. cruzi - T. gambiense - T. rhodesiense	 - American trypanosomiasis (Chagas) - kissing bug *- Rx : nifurtimox* - Tsetse fly : - African sleeping sickness - more severe than gambiense *- Rx : suramin, melarsoprol*

2.32.) <u>INTESTINAL PROTOZOA</u>

Entamoeba histolytica	- cysts have 4 nuclei - bloody, mucus, diarrhea - liver abscess - can be sexually transmitted - *Rx : metronidazole*
Giardia lamblia	- cyst: 4 nuclei - trophozoite: 2 nuclei, 4 pairs of flagella (looks like a clown....) - excystation in duodenum - nonbloody, foul smelling diarrhea - *Rx : metronidazole*
Cryptosporidium	- excystation in small intestine - trophozoites do not invade gut wall - severe diarrhea in immunocompromised - *no effective therapy*

<u>another protozoon just for comparison :</u>

Trichomonas	- 1 nucleus, 4 flagella, undulating membrane - most common VD in the US ! - male : non-purulent urethritis or asymptomatic - female: foul-smelling, watery, green discharge - *Rx : metronidazole*

2.33.) <u>TREMATODES (FLUKES)</u>

Sch. mansoni	penetrates skin	veins of colon
Sch. japonicum	penetrates skin	veins of small intestine
Sch. hematobium	penetrates skin	veins of urinary bladder
Clonorchis sinensis	raw fish	liver
Paragonimus	raw crab meat	lung

Rx : Praziquantel

2.34.) CESTODES (TAPEWORMS)

T. solium	pork	larvae	intestine
T. solium	human feces	eggs	cysticerci (in brain, eyes)
T. saginata	beef	larvae	intestine
D. latum	raw fish	larvae	intestine
Echinococcus	dog feces	eggs	cysts (in liver, lung, brain)

Rx : Niclosamide

2.35.) NEMATODES (ROUNDWORMS)

Enterobius[1]	perianal pruritus (at night)
Ascaris[1]	worm lives in colon, larves migrate to lung
Necator[2]	intestinal blood loss
Strongyloides[2]	larves penetrate skin, then migrate to lung
Trichinella[2]	pork meat, larvae form cysts in striated muscle
Wucheria[3]	microfilariae found in blood adult worm lives in lymphnodes -> lymph. obstruction
Onchocerca[3]	"river blindness" microfilariae in subcutaneous tissue and eye

[1]ingested eggs
[2]larvae
[3]insect bite

2.36.) <u>COMPLEMENT</u>

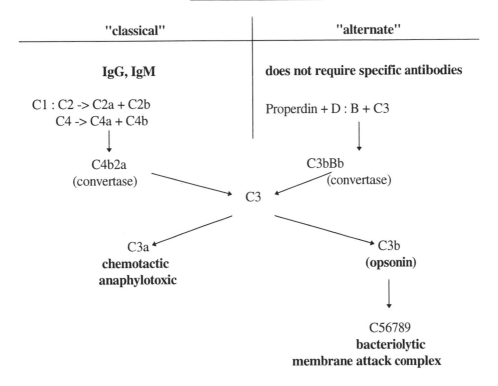

"classical"	"alternate"
IgG, IgM	does not require specific antibodies

C1 : C2 -> C2a + C2b
C4 -> C4a + C4b

Properdin + D : B + C3

C4b2a
(convertase)

C3bBb
(convertase)

C3

C3a
**chemotactic
anaphylotoxic**

C3b
(opsonin)

C56789
**bacteriolytic
membrane attack complex**

2.37.) <u>MEDIATORS OF INFLAMMATION</u>

fever	IL-1, PG
vasodilatation	histamine, bradykinin, lymphokines, PGE
exudation	histamine, bradykinin
chemotaxis	lymphokines, PG2α, C5a
phagocytosis	lymphokines, C3b
pain	PG, bradykinin

2.38.) FAMOUS SEROLOGICAL TESTS

(mainly of historical interest)

	Test	Principle	read as "+"	false positives
Rickettsia	Weil-Felix	agglutination with Proteus antigens	if agglutination occurs	- proteus UTI - leptospirosis - liver diseases
Salmonella	Widal	agglutination[*]	if agglutination occurs	- normal (1:10) - other crossreacting gram - rods
Treponema	Wassermann	complement fixation	if sensitized RBC lysis does not occur	- yaws - malaria - pregnancy

* formalinized : H-antibodies (anti flagellar)
  alcoholized : O-antibodies (anti surface)

PHARMACOLOGY

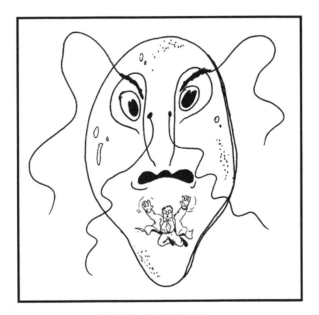

Antibiotic failures.

3.1.) <u>DRUG INTERACTIONS</u>

drugs that are easily displaced from albumins	sulfonamides phenylbutazone tolbutamide coumarins
drugs that induce P450	alcohol barbiturates phenytoin rifampicin
drugs that inhibit P450	chloramphenicol cimetidine phenylbutazone
drugs that compete for renal transporters	(uric acid) probenecid penicillins sulfonamides salicylates thiazides

3.2.) <u>ANTIDOTES</u>

acetaminophen	N-acetylcysteine
opiates	naloxone
benzodiazepines	flumazenil
methanol	ethanol
CO	O_2
cyanide	amylnitrate
organophosphates	atropine, pralidoxime
iron	deferoxamine

3.3.) <u>ANTIBIOTICS</u>

bactericidal	bacteriostatic
penicillins	chloramphenicol
cephalosporins	erythromycin
aminoglycosides	tetracyclines
vancomycin	sulfonamides
	trimethoprim

3.4.) <u>PENICILLINS</u>

narrow spectrum **β-lactamase sensitive**	penicillin G penicillin V	gram positive strept.
β-lactamase resistant	methicillin oxacillin nafcillin cloxacillin	gram positive strept.
broad spectrum	ampicillin amoxicillin	Hemophilus Neisseria E. coli Proteus
extended spectrum	carbenicillin	Pseudomonas

3.5.) <u>CEPHALOSPORINS</u>

1st Generation

cefazolin	longest half life
cephopirin	most resistant to β-lactamase

2nd Generation

cefamandole	anti vit. K disulfiram like reaction with ethanol
cefotetan	best against anaerobes
cefotixin	best against anaerobes

3rd Generation

cefotaxime	CNS permeable
ceftriaxone	for penicillin resistant gonorrhea

3.6.) <u>ANTI-VIRAL</u>

amantadine	impairs uncoating	influenza A
ribavirin	guanosine analog	RSV infections in children
acyclovir	guanine analog, depends on viral thymidine kinase	HSV-1, HSV-2, VZV
vidarabine	adenosine analog	all Herpes group viruses
idoxuridine	thymidine analog	herpes simplex keratitis
ganciclovir	like acyclovir	for CMV
AZT[1]	thymidine analog	for HIV
interferon	glycoprotein inhibits viral multiplication	leukemia Kaposi sarcoma genital warts hepatitis B and C

[1] 3'-azido-3'-deoxythymidine

3.7.) ANTI-FUNGAL AND PROTOZOA

leishmaniasis	stibugluconate
systemic fungal infections	amphotericin B
candida, skin, GI	nystatin
broad spectrum anti-fungals	imidazoles
dermatophytic Infections	griseofulvin

malaria : a) prophylaxis
          b) therapy
          b) therapy (p.falciparum)
          c) prevention of relapse
	mefloquine
	chloroquine
	quinine + pyrimethamine/sulfadoxine
	primaquine

amebiasis (Trichomonas, Chlamydia)	metronidazole
Trypanosoma gambiense **Trypanosoma rhodesiense** (African sleeping sickness)	melarsoprol / suramine
Trypanosoma cruzi (Chagas disease)	nifurtimox

3.8.) DRUGS OF CHOICE

Actinomyces	actinomycosis	penicillin G
Bacillus anthracis	anthrax	penicillin G
Bordetella pertussis	whooping cough	erythromycin
Borrelia Burgdorferi	Lyme disease	tetracycline
Campylobacter	acute inflammatory diarrhea	quinolones
Candida[1]	candidiasis	fluconazole
Chlamydia	pneumonia	tetracyclin
	lymphgranuloma venerum	doxycyclin
H. influenza	pneumonia, meningitis	3rd gen. cephalosporin
Helicobacter pylori	gastric ulcer	metronidazole + tetracycline
Klebsiella	pneumonia	3rd gen. cephalosporin
	UTI	quinolones
		trimethoprim/sulfamethoxazole
Legionella	Legionnaire's disease	erythromycin
M. tuberculosis	tuberculosis	isoniazide + rifampin
		("2nd line" : cycloserine)
M. leprae	leprosy	dapsone + rifampin
M. pneumoniae	atypical pneumonia	erythromycin
N. gonorrhea	gonorrhea	ceftriaxone
N. meningitis	meningitis	penicillin G
Nocardia	pneumonia	trimethoprim/sulfamethoxazole
Proteus	UTI	quinolones
Rickettsia	spotted fever, end. typhus	doxycycline
Salmonella typhi	typhoid fever	trimethoprim/sulfamethoxazole
Shigella		trimethoprim/sulfamethoxazole
Staph. aureus	skin infection	methicillin
	otitis, sinusitis	amoxicillin-clavulinate
Strept. pyogenes	pharyngitis, erysipelas	penicillin G or V
Strept. viridans	endocarditis	penicillin + aminoglycoside
Treponema pallidum	syphilis	penicillin G
Trichomonas[2]	trichomoniasis	metronidazole
Tropheryma whippelii	Whipple's disease	trimethoprim/sulfamethoxazole
Vibrio cholerae	cholera	tetracycline
Yersinia pestis	plague ("black death")	streptomycin

[1] a yeast, [2] a protozoon

3.9.) __AIDS-RELATED__

HIV	zidovudine (AZT)
HSV	acyclovir
CMV	ganciclovir
Mycobacterium tuberculosis	isoniazid-rifampin (cycloserine if resistant)
Candida	clotrimazole
Cryptococcus neoformans	amphotericin B
Pneumocystis carinii	trimethoprim-sulfamethoxasole (pentamidine if allergic)
Toxoplasma gondii	pyrimethamine-sulfadiazine

3.10.) <u>ANTI-NEOPLASTIC</u>
(indications)

Wilms	dactinomycin vinblastine
Hodgkin	mechlorethamine vincristine prednisone procarbazine
testicular tumors	bleomycin vinblastine cisplatin
ALL	prednisone vincristine

3.11.) <u>ANTI-NEOPLASTIC</u>
(specific side effects)

doxorubicin	cardiotoxic
cyclophosphamide	hemorrhagic cystitis
bleomycin	pneumonitis
vincristine	periph. neuropathy
cisplatin	renal toxicity
L-asparaginase	allergic reactions

<u>Cycle-specific</u> :
antimetabolites, bleomycin, vinca alkaloids

115

3.12.) NSAIDs

aspirin	- irreversibly acetylates cyclo oxygenase	- analgesic: 600 mg/d - anti-inflammatory: 4g/d - may cause Reye's syndrome - contraindicated in gout !
acetaminophen	- no anti-inflammatory action - prefers CNS cyclo oxygenase	- DOC for children with viral infections
ibuprofen	- similar spectrum as aspirin	- fewer GI side-effects
phenylbutazone	- anti-inflammatory - weak analgesic/antipyretic	- used when others have failed - may cause skin rash, GI upset
indomethacin	- more potent anti-inflammatory than aspirin	- for acute gout - for ankylosing spondylitis - may cause GI, CNS, pancreatitis
gold	- suppresses macrophages	- for rheumatoid arthritis - not for acute attack
D-penicillamine	- reduces rheumatoid factor	- for rheumatoid arthritis - when gold has failed - also chelates heavy metals
methotrexate	- folic acid antagonist (much lower dose used than for cancer therapy)	- for severe rheumatoid arthritis - when all else has failed - may cause cytopenia

3.13.) <u>GOUT</u>

acute	**colchicine**	- inhibits migration of macrophages (depolymerizes microtubules)
chronic	**allopurinol**	- purine analog - inhibits xanthine oxidase
chronic	**probenecid**	- blocks tubular secretion of penicillin - blocks tubular reabsorption of uric acid

3.14.) ANTI-HYPERTENSIVES

	indications	contraindications
β-blockers	- angina pectoris - post MI	- diabetes - asthma - peripheral vascular disease
diuretics	- congestive heart failure - chronic renal failure	- diabetes - hyperlipidemia
Ca^{2+} channel blockers	- for all	- congestive heart failure
ACE inhibitors	- for all	- pregnancy

3.15.) ANTI-ANGIOTENSINS

captopril	- ACE inhibitor - decreases angiotensin II - increases bradykinin
enalapril	- ACE inhibitor - more potent - longer half time
saralazin	- blocks angiotensin receptors (weak agonist)

3.16.) ERGOT ALKALOIDS

ergotamine methysergide	vasoconstriction	- for migraine - post partum hemorrhage
bromocriptine	inhibits prolactin release	- for hyperprolactinemia (pituitary adenomas) - for infertility

3.17.) DIURETICS

carb. anhydrase inhibitors	acetazolamide	- weak - rarely used	- metabolic acidosis
loop diuretics	furosemide ethacrynic acid	- acute pulmonary edema - hypercalcemia	- ototoxicity - hypokalemia - hyperuricemia
thiazides	chlorothiazide hydrochlorothiazide chlorthalidone	- hypertension - mild congestive heart failure - urinary Ca stones - diabetes insipidus	- hypokalemia - hypercalcemia - hyperglycemia - hyperuricemia
potassium sparing	spironolactone (aldosterone antagonist) amiloride triamterene	- usually combined with thiazides or loop diuretics - secondary hyperaldosteronism	- spironolactone does not work in Addison's ! - amiloride and triamterene do not depend on aldosterone
osmotic diuretics	mannitol	- acute renal failure - not for conditions a/w Na^+ retention	

3.18.) <u>ANTI-ANGINAL</u>

nitroglycerin	- low dose : dilates veins, reduces preload - high dose: also dilates arterioles, reflex tachycardia (angina may get worse)
isosorbide dinitrate	- orally active - less potent than nitroglycerine
nifedipine	- relaxes arterioles - best for Prinzmetal's angina (coronary artery spasm)
verapamil	- slows heart rate - effect partially overcome by reflex tachycardia

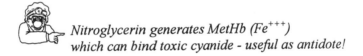

Nitroglycerin generates MetHb (Fe^{+++})
which can bind toxic cyanide - useful as antidote!

3.19.) __PLATELET AGGREGATION INHIBITORS__

aspirin	- inhibits cycloxygenase (block of thromboxane synthesis)
sulfinpyrazone	- inhibits degranulation - also prolongs survival of platelets

dipyridamole	- PDE inhibitor
	- increases cAMP and
	  inhibits degranulation
	  (serotonin, ADP)

3.20.) __ANTICOAGULANTS__

		Antagonist
heparin	- enhances activity of antithrombin III	protamine sulfate
warfarin **dicumarol**	- antagonist of vit. K (II, VII, IX, X)	vit. K
streptokinase	- made from group C streptococci - activates plasminogen - plasmin degrades fibrin	aminocaproic acid
urokinase	- made from human fetal renal cells - less antigenicity than streptokinase	

TPA	- "fibrin selective"
	  (activates only plasminogen
	  already bound to fibrin)	

3.21.) ANTI-ARRHYTHMICS

		action potential	upstroke velocity	
1A	quinidine	↑	↓	- inhibits ectopic arrythmias potentiates digitoxin !
	procainamide			- inhibits ectopic arrythmias - reversible lupus erythematosus
1B	lidocaine	↓	↓	- acute ventricular flutter/fibrill. - digitalis induced arrhythmias
	phenytoin			- same gingiva hyperplasia
1C	flecainide encainide	∅	↓	- "broad spectrum"
2	propanolol			- atrial tachycardia - post MI (prophylactic)
3	bretylium amiodarone			- severe unresponsive ventricular arrhythmias
4	verapamil			- atrial tachicardia - atrial flutter

class 1	Na$^+$ channel blockers
class 2	β-blockers
class 3	K$^+$ channel blockers
class 4	Ca^{2+} channel blockers

3.22.) __INOTROPICS__

glycosides[1]	**digoxin** **digitoxin**	- low therapeutic index - decreased AV conduction - tachycardia, fibrillations - hypokalemia potentiates toxicity - digoxin: short, digitoxin: long action
β-agonists	**dobutamine** **(dopamine)**	- increase cAMP - less tachycardia or peripheral side effects than isoproterenol or epinephrine
PDE inhibitors	**amrinone** **milrinone**	- thrombocytopenia - does not affect platelets

[1] *__toxicity of glycosides is enhanced by__ :*
hypokalemia
alkalosis
hypoxia
hypothyroidism

3.23.) <u>ASTHMA</u>

mild, intermittent	**metaproterenol** **terbutaline** **albuterol**
more severe	**theophylline** (caveat: seizures, arrhythmias)
prophylaxis	**cromolyn**
chronic, and status asthmaticus	**corticosteroids**

3.24.) <u>INSULINS</u>

		Peak	Duration
CZI	- "regular insulin" - IV (only soluble prep.)	30 min	120 min
semilente	- given subcutaneously - rapid onset	2-3 h	5-8 h
lente	- mix of semi and ultra	8-12 h	18-24 h
ultralente	- prolonged action	14-20 h	36 h
PZI	- CZI treated with protamine	14-20 h	36 h

3.25.) <u>SULFONYLUREAS</u>

	Duration
tolbutamide	8 h
glyburide **glipizide**	20 h, most potent
chlorpropamide	48 h

126

3.26.) <u>HYPERLIPIDEMIAS I</u>

Type I	chylomicrons *TGA*	lipoprotein lipase
Type IIA	LDL *cholesterol*	LDL receptor
Type IIB	LDL *cholesterol* VLDL *TGA*	LDL receptor
Type III	IDL *TGA* *cholesterol*	mutant apoprotein ?
Type IV	VLDL *TGA*	overproduction (liver) or underutilization

3.27.) <u>HYPERLIPIDEMIAS II</u>

diet	- helps all - only option for type I	I
niacin	- inhibits lipolysis in fat cells - decreases free fatty acids (decreased VLDL synthesis)	IIB

clofibrate	- activates lipoprotein lipase
	   (increases VLDL utilization)
	- inhibits cholesterol synthesis
	- enhances cholesterol excretion in bile
	   (may promote gallbladder stones)
		III and IV

cholestyramine **colestipol**	- anion exchanger (binds cholesterol in gut)	IIA, IIB
lovastatin	- inhibits HMG-CoA reductase	IIA, IIB

3.28.) __PEPTIC ULCERS__

H$_2$ blockers	**- cimetidine**	- anti-androgenic
	- ranitidine	- more potent, longer acting no anti-androgenic action
	- famotidine	- most potent
prostaglandins	**- misoprostol**	- analog of PGE
proton pump inhibitors	**- omeprazol**	- drug of choice !
anti muscarinic	**- pirenzepine**	- reduces acid secretion - less effect on motility - usually combined with others
antacids	**- Al (OH)$_3$** **- Mg (OH)$_3$**	- may cause constipation - may cause diarrhea
mucosa protection	**- bismuth** **- sucralfate**	

3.29.) ADRENERGIC

α-blockers	phenoxybenzamine	α1 , α2, irreversible	- autonomic hyperreflexia
	phentolamine	α1 , α2, reversible	- hypertensive crisis
	prazosin	α1	- hypertension
α-agonists	phenylephrine	α1	- nasal decongestant
	methoxamine	α1	- hypotension
	clonidine	α2 , central	- hypertension
β-blockers	propanolol	β1 , β2	⎫ hypertension
	pindolol	β1 , β2 + ISA	⎬ migraine (prophyl.)
	metoprolol	β1	⎭ glaucoma
	atenolol	β1	
	labetalol	β , α	
β-agonists	isoproterenol	β1 , β2	- bronchospasm
	metaproterenol	β2	- bronchospasm
	dobutamine	β1	- congestive heart failure
	dopamine	D1 > β1	- shock
indirect -	reserpine	deplete stores	⎫ hypertension
	guanethidine		⎭
indirect +	ephedrine	prolong action	- nasal decongestant
	amphetamine		- narcolepsy, ADHD

3.30.) CHOLINESTERASE INHIBITORS

physostigmine	- may cause convulsions
neostigmine	- does not enter CNS - better action on skeletal muscle
edrophonium	- shortest duration of action
organophosphates	- irreversible - pralidoxime prevents aging

3.31.) DIRECT CHOLINERGIC

bethanechol	- atonic bladder / GI	muscarinic
pilocarpine	- less potent - acute glaucoma	muscarinic
carbachol	- not hydrolyzed	muscarinic and nicotinic

3.32.) ANTI-MUSCARINIC

atropine	- anti-spasmodic - mydriasis - organophosphate poisoning
scopolamine	- greater CNS action - for motion sickness

3.33.) ANTI-NICOTINIC

tubocurarine	- blocks nicotinic ACh receptor
pancuronium	- less histamine release than tubocurarine
gallamine	- less histamine release than tubocurarine
succinyl choline	- depolarizing - very short duration of action - for malignant hyperthermia : dantolene

 drugs that enhance neuromuscular block :
halothane
aminoglycosides
Ca^{2+} channel blockers

3.34.) SEX-HORMONES

ESTROGENS	PROGESTERONES
nausea vomiting breast tenderness skin pigmentation hypertension breakthrough bleeding	weight gain depression hirsutism
oral contraceptive **"morning after pill"** hormone replacement	oral contraceptive **"mini pill"** habitual abortion endometriosis

 __Risks of Oral Contraceptives__

- *thromboemboli*
- *benign adenoma of the liver*
- *vaginal cancers in daughters of mothers who received DES*

- ***but not*** *: breast cancer or endometrial cancer*

3.35.) <u>HALLUCINOGENS</u>

LSD	- acts on 5-HT_1 and 5-HT_2 receptors - activates sympathetic system - brilliant color hallucinations (blockable by neuroleptics) - may trigger psychosis
THC	- enhanced sensory activity - impaired mental activity - impaired short term memory - red conjunctivas
PCP	- reuptake inhibitor - dissociative anesthesia - bizarre and hostile behavior

3.36.) <u>OPIOIDS</u>

mu	**morphine** **met-enkephalin**	euphoria, dependence analgesia respiratory depression
delta	**leu-enkephalin**	mood changes
kappa	**dynorphin**	analgesia, miosis, sedation
sigma	**pentazocine**	dysphoria, hallucinations respiratory stimulation

naloxone	- μ, κ, σ antagonist
pentazocine	- κ, σ agonist - δ, (μ) antagonist
codeine	- weak analgesic (like aspirin) - good antitussive - low abuse potential
propoxyphene	- dextro : analgesic - levo : antitussive
fentanyl	- 80x potency of morphine
methadone	- longer duration of action than morphine - used for controlled withdrawal

3.37.) <u>ANTI-DEPRESSANTS</u>

TCA : amitryptiline amoxapine desipramine etc.	- block uptake (NE, serotonin, dopa.) - block receptors (m, α, serotonin, hist.)	- slow onset of action - inconsistent bioavailability
imipramine		- for enuresis
"Next Generation" **fluoxetine** **trazodone**	- selectively block uptake of serotonin	- fewer anticholinergic effects
MAO inhibitors	- increases amount of transmitter stored	- "second choice" - have stimulant properties - caveat : tyramine !
lithium	- treat manic episodes - prophylaxis for manic and depressed episodes	- low therapeutic index - excreted by kidney - ataxia, tremors confusion, convulsions

3.38.) <u>CNS STIMULANTS</u>

methylxanthines	**caffeine** **theophylline**	- low dose : increased alertness - high dose : anxiety, tremors - smooth muscle relaxation - weak diuretic - enhanced HCl secretion in stomach
others	**nicotine**	- low dose : ganglion stimulating, BP↑ - high dose: ganglion blockade, BP ↓
	cocaine	- reuptake inhibitor - local anesthetic and vasoconstrictor - euphoria, hallucinations delusions, paranoia - cardiac arrythmias
	amphetamine	- release of stored catecholamines - effects like cocaine - euphoria lasts longer than cocaine - no tolerance to CNS toxicity

3.39.) ANXIOLYTIC

benzodiazepines	diazepam	- long acting - for status epilepticus
	chlordiazepoxide	- long acting - for alcohol withdrawal
	lorazepam triazolam	- short acting - more severe withdrawal symptoms
others	buspirone	- acts on 5-HT$_{1A}$ receptors - slow onset of action - little sedation - little dependence

3.40.) HYPNOTIC

barbiturates	phenobarbital	- long acting, for seizures
	thiopental	- short acting, for anesthesia
others	chloralhydrate	- for children, causes epigastric pain
	meprobamate	- less sedation, better anxiolytic

3.41.) H₁ BLOCKERS

diphenhydramine [1] **doxylamine** **promethazine**	sedation
meclizine [1] **timeprazine**	long half life
terfenadine **aztenazole**	non-sedating, but very slow onset of action

[1] for motion sickness

3.42.) ANESTHETICS

MAC : N_2O > ether > enflurane > halothane
onset : N_2O > enflurane > halothane > ether

Inhalation

halothane	- lacks analgesic potency - hepatotoxic for adults - cardiac arrythmias - malignant hyperthermia
enflurane	- excreted by kidney rather than liver
isoflurane	- does not induce arrythmias - lower toxicity
N_2O	- not potent - does not depress respiration - safe

I.V.

thiopental	- ultrashort barbiturate - not analgesic
ketamine	- dissociative anesthesia (patient appears awake but is unconscious) - post op. hallucinations

Examples:

balanced anesthesia : thiopental + fentanyl + tubocurarine + N_2O
neurolept anesthesia : droperidol + fentanyl + N_2O

3.43.) **PARKINSON**

dopaminergic	**levodopa plus carbidopa**	- CNS permeable - inhibits peripheral decarboxylase
	bromocriptine	- direct dopamine agonist
	deprenyl	- inhibits MAO-B (dopamine selective)
	amantadine	- enhances dopamine metabolism
anticholinergic	**benztropine biperiden**	- secondary drugs

3.44.) NEUROLEPTICS

phenothiazine	chlorpromazine	- anticholinergic side effects - arrythmias - rarely used
	fluphenazine	- long acting - for outpatients
butyrophenone	haloperidol	- extrapyramidal side effects - fewer anticholinergic side effects
	droperidol	- for neurolept anesthesia
other	clozapine	- fewer extrapyramidal side effects - bone marrow suppression

3.45.) ANTI-EMETIC

motion sickness	scopolamine
vertigo	meclizine
chemotherapy	metoclopramide diphenhydramine
radiation therapy	domperidone

3.46.) ANTI-EPILEPTIC

partial focal	**phenytoin, carbamazepine**
grand mal	**phenytoin, carbamazepine**
petit mal	**ethosuximide** **phenytoin is contraindicated !**
myoclonic	**valproic acid, clonazepam**
febrile seizures (children)	**phenobarbital**
status epilepticus	**diazepam, phenytoin**

BIOCHEMISTRY

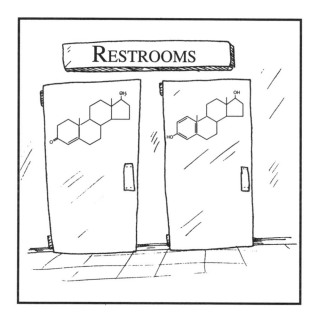

4.1.) <u>AMINO ACIDS</u>

acidic	Asp, Glu
basic	His, Lys, Arg
essential	Ile, Val, Leu Try, Phe, Met Lys, Arg, His, Thr
ketogenic	Leu, Lys (Phe, Trp, Tyr)

trypsin cleaves at	Arg, Lys
chemotrypsin cleaves at	Phe, Tyr, Trp

4.2.) <u>AMINO ACID PRECURSORS</u>

tyrosine	- dopa, dopamine - norepinephrine, epinephrine - T_3, T_4 (thyroxin) - melanin
tryptophan	- 5-HT (serotonin) - melatonin - niacin
glutamate	- GABA
glycine	- porphyrin, heme - creatine (gly + arg)
histidine	- histamine

4.3.) <u>AMINO ACID DISORDERS</u>

phenylketonuria	phenylalanine hydroxylase	- mental retardation - hypopigmentation - musty odor
alkaptonuria	homogentisate oxidase	- arthritis (ochronosis) - urine darkens
maple syrup	branched chain dehydrogenase	- hyperreflexia - sweet odor
homocystinuria	cystathione synthetase	- mental retardation - lens dislocation
cystinuria	dibasic amino acid transporter	- cystine calculi

hartnup disease	neutral amino acid transporter	- tryptophan deficiency
		   -> niacin deficiency
		   -> pellagra

4.4.) <u>HEXOSES</u>

<u>epimers</u>

β	CHO α	<u>glucose</u>	<u>mannose</u>	<u>galactose</u>
	2-OH	R	L	R
OH-3		L	L	L
	4-OH	R	R	L
L	5-OH D			
	CH₂OH			

pyranose	- ring with 5 carbons + 1 oxygen
furanose	- ring with 4 carbons + 1 oxygen
anomeric carbon	- C atoms that have 4 different ligands - usually refers to C1 in ring form
epimers	- isomers that differ in only one carbon (e.g. glucose and galactose)
enantiomers	- mirror image (i.e. flipped at all anomeric carbons)
reducing sugars	- if oxygen on carbonyl group (C1) is available for redox (e.g. glucose, fructose but not sucrose)

4.5.) <u>SACCHARIDES</u>

maltose	glucose + glucose	α1-4
lactose	galactose + glucose	β1-4
sucrose	glucose + fructose	α1-β2 (non-reducing !)
glycogen, starch	many glucoses	α1-4 and α1-6
cellulose	many glucoses	β1-4

4.6.) <u>SACCHARIDE DISORDERS</u>

fructosuria	fructokinase	- benign - asymptomatic
fructose intolerance	aldolase B	- hypoglycemia - liver failure
galactosemia	galactokinase or uridyltransferase	- cataracts - mental retardation
lactose intolerance	lactase (usually acquired)	- diarrhea

4.7.) <u>GLYCOGEN STORAGE</u>

Type I von Gierke	glucose-6-phosphatase[1]	- liver, kidney, intestine
Type II Pompe	α-glucosidase (lysosomes)	- generalized
Type V McArdle	sk. muscle phosphorylase	- muscle weakness

 [1]*skeletal muscle cells don't have this enzyme*

4.8.) <u>GLYCOSAMINOGLYCANS</u>

Hurler	α-L Iduronidase[2]	- cornea clouding - mental retardation
Scheie	α-L Iduronidase[2]	- cornea clouding - normal intelligence
Hunter	Iduronate sulfatase	- no clouding - mental retardation

 [2]*different mutations!*

150

4.9.) <u>FATTY ACIDS</u>

palmitic	16:0	**stearic**	18:0
palmitoleic	16:1(9)	**oleic**	18:1(9)
linoleic	18:2(9,12)	**arachidonic**	20:4(5,8,11,14)
linolenic	18:3(9,12,15)		

4.10.) <u>BILE ACIDS</u>

primary	- cholic acid - chenodeoxycholic acid
secondary	- deoxycholic acid - lithocholic acid

conjugates	- glycocholic acid
	  (cholic acid + glycine)
	
	- taurocholic acid
	  (cholic acid + taurine)
	
	etc...

4.11.) <u>PHOSPHOLIPIDS</u>

A) <u>Glycerols</u>

phosphatidyl choline (lecithin)	phosphatidic acid + choline
phosphatidyl ethanolamine	phosphatidic acid + ethanolamine
phosphatidyl serine	phosphatidic acid + serine
phosphatidyl inositol	phosphatidic acid + inositol
cardiolipin	2x phosphatidic acid + glycerine

B) <u>Sphingosines</u>

ceramide	sphingosine + any fatty acid
sphingomyelin	ceramide + choline

4.12.) <u>GLYCOLIPIDS</u>

C) <u>More Sphingosines</u>

cerebroside	ceramide mono saccharide
globoside	ceramide oligo saccharide
ganglioside	ceramide oligo saccharide + NANA

4.13.) <u>SPHINGOLIPIDOSES</u>

Niemann-Pick	A	sphingomyelin	- liver and spleen enlargement - foamy cells
Gaucher	A	glucocerebrosides	- liver and spleen enlargement - osteoporosis - Ashkenazic jews
Krabbe	A	galactocerebrosides	- blindness, deafness - convulsions - globoid cells
metachromatic l.	A	sulfatides	- progressive paralysis
Fabry	X	globosides	- reddish/purple skin rash - kidney/heart failure - angiokeratoma
Tay-Sachs	A	gangliosides	- blindness - cherry red maculas - Ashkenazic jews

A: Autosomal recessive
X: X-linked recessive

4.14.) PORPHYRIAS

acute intermittent	porphobilinogen	- urine is photosensitive - patients are not
cutanea tarda	uroporphobilinogen	- patients are photosensitive - most common
coproporphyria	coproporphyrinogen	- patients are photosensitive

lead poisoning	coproporphyrinogen
	ALA
		- anemia
		  microcytic, hypochromic
		  "basophil stippling"

4.15.) <u>PREFERRED NUTRIENTS</u>

brain	- glucose (usually) - ketone bodies (when starved)
muscle	- glucose (when working) - fatty acids (when resting)
heart	- ketone bodies - (glucose)
erythrocytes	- glucose

4.16.) <u>VITAMINS</u>

A	- night blindness (retinal) - growth retardation (retinoic acid)	- part of rhodopsine
D	- rickets, osteomalacia	- intest. Ca^{2+} absorption - bone : supports PTH
E	- ataxia	- anti oxidant
K	- bleeding-disorder (II, VII, IX, X)	- **carboxylation** of glutamate
C	- scurvy	- hydroxylation of proline and lysine
B1 (thiamin)	- beriberi	- **decarboxylations**
B2 (riboflavin)	- glossitis, cheilosis	- flavins (FMN etc.)
B6 (pyridoxin)	- anemia (microcytic) - neuropathy	- **transaminations** - **deaminations**
B12	- anemia (macrocytic) - neuropathy - *D. Latum* !	- methionine synthesis - odd carbon FA degrad.
niacin	- pellagra (diarrhea, dementia, dermatitis)	- NAD^+, NADPH
pantothenate	- headache, nausea	- CoA
biotin	- seborrhoic dermatitis - nervous disorders - *avidin* !	- **carboxylations**
folic acid	- anemia (macrocytic) - glossitis, colitis	- one carbon metabolism

4.17.) <u>ATP EQUIVALENTS</u>

FADH$_2$	2	
NADH	3	
acetyl CoA	12	acetyl CoA -> 2 CO$_2$ 3 NADH + FADH$_2$ + GTP
pyruvate	15	pyruvate -> acetyl CoA + NADH
glycolysis (anaerobe)	2	glucose -> lactate 4 ATP - 2 ATP
glycolysis (aerobe)	8	glucose -> pyruvate (4 ATP - 2 ATP) + 2 NADH
glucose (complete oxidation)	38	glucose -> 6 CO$_2$ 8 + 2x15 (pyruvate)
fatty acid (e.g. 16:0)	129	
gluconeogenesis (from pyruvate)	-12	
urea synthesis	-4	

 NADH gives only 2 ATP if glycerophosphate shuttle instead of malate shuttle is used.

157

4.18.) KEY ENZYMES

	enzyme	-	+	phosphorylation
glycolysis	phosphofructokinase 1	ATP citrate	AMP fructose 2,6 -dp	inhibits
	phosphofructokinase 2			
gluconeogenesis	fructosediphosphatase 1		ATP citrate	activates
	fructosediphosphatase 2	AMP fructose 2,6 -dp		
glycogenolysis	glycogenphosphorylase			activates
glycogen synthesis	glycogen synthetase			inhibits
pentose phosphate shunt	glucose-6-phosphate dehydrogenase	NADPH		

- : allosteric inhibitor
+: allosteric activator

4.19.) MORE KEY ENZYMES

	enzyme	−	+	phosphorylation
lipolysis	carnitine acyltransferase	malonyl CoA		
fat mobilization	hormone sensitive lipase			activates
lipid synthesis	acetyl-CoA carboxylase		citrate	inhibits
cholesterol synthesis	HMG CoA reductase		cholesterol	inhibits

− : allosteric inhibitor
+: allosteric activator

4.20.) __EVEN MORE KEY ENZYMES__

	enzyme	–	phosphorylation
ketone body synthesis	HMG CoA synthase		
purine synthesis	amidotransferase	AMP GMP IMP	
citric acid cycle	pyruvate dehydrogenase		inhibits Acetyl CoA ATP NADH

– : allosteric inhibitor

160

4.21.) <u>HEXOSE KINASES</u>

	Hexokinase	Glucokinase
tissues	many	liver, β-cells
substrate specificity	hexoses	same !
affinity	high	low
V_{max} ("capacity")	low	high
inhibited by glucose-6-phosphate	yes	no

4.22.) <u>STEROIDS</u>

Class	Example	C-atoms
sterols	cholesterol	27
bile acids	glycocholate taurocholate	24
adrenal steroids	cortisol aldosterone	21
gestogens	progesterone	21
androgens	testosterone, androstenedione	19
estrogens	estradiol	18

17 ketosteroids   : androgens except testosterone
17 hydroxysteroids : cortisol metabolites

4.23.) <u>ADRENAL GLAND</u>

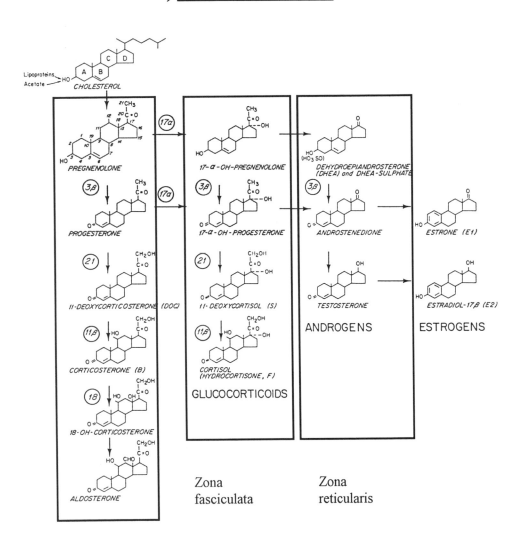

Zona
glomerulosa

Zona
fasciculata

Zona
reticularis

4.24.) <u>TESTIS (Leydig Cells)</u>

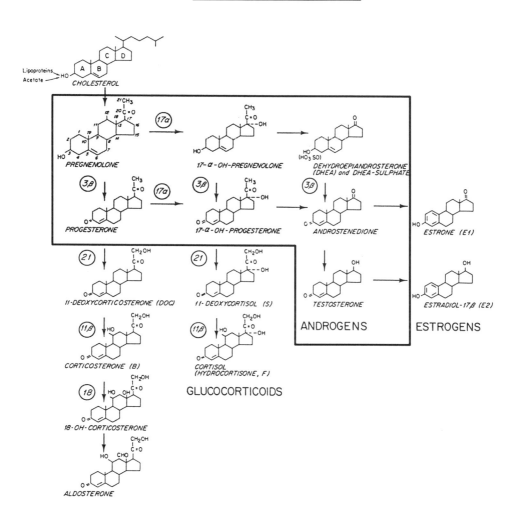

CHOLESTEROL

PREGNENOLONE

17-α-OH-PREGNENOLONE

DEHYDROEPIANDROSTERONE
(DHEA) and DHEA-SULPHATE

PROGESTERONE

17-α-OH-PROGESTERONE

ANDROSTENEDIONE

ESTRONE (E1)

11-DEOXYCORTICOSTERONE (DOC)

11-DEOXYCORTISOL (S)

TESTOSTERONE

ESTRADIOL-17β (E2)

ANDROGENS

ESTROGENS

CORTICOSTERONE (B)

CORTISOL
(HYDROCORTISONE, F)

18-OH-CORTICOSTERONE

GLUCOCORTICOIDS

ALDOSTERONE

164

4.25.) <u>PERIPHERAL METABOLISM</u>

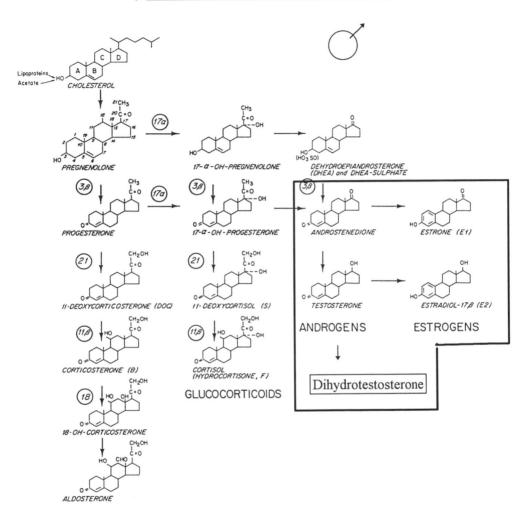

165

4.26.) OVARY (Theca Cells)

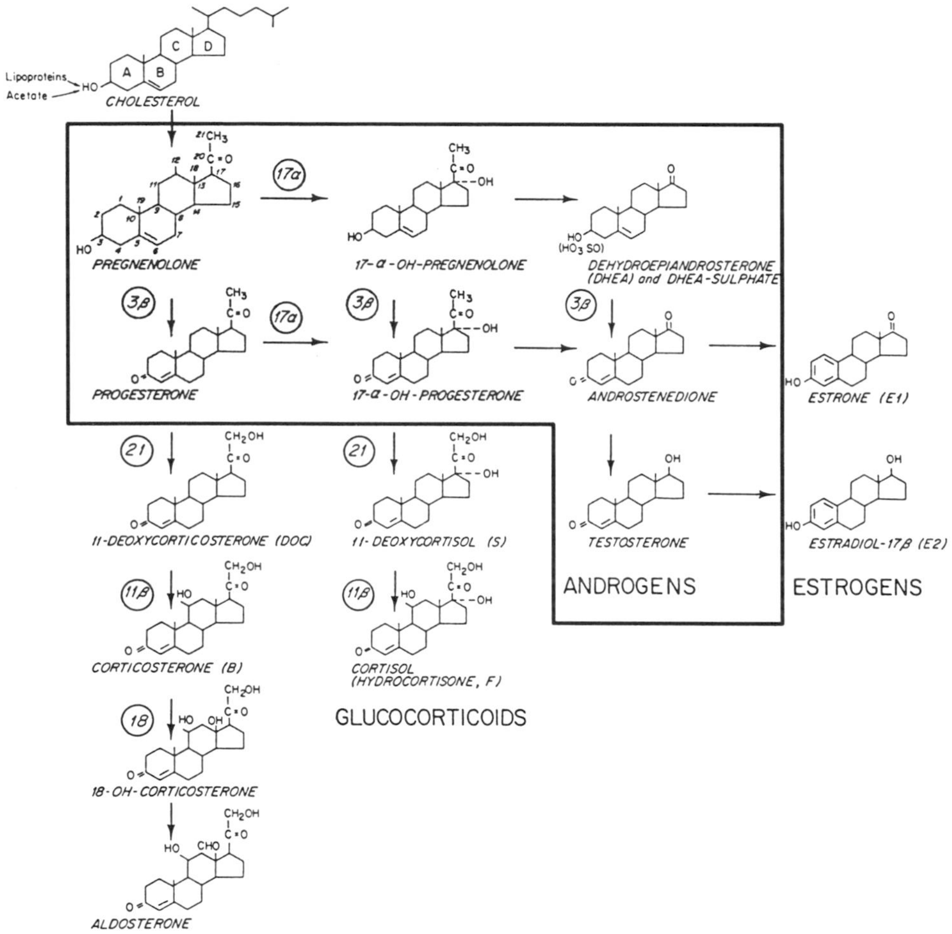

Lipoproteins
Acetate
CHOLESTEROL
PREGNENOLONE
17α
17-α-OH-PREGNENOLONE
DEHYDROEPIANDROSTERONE (DHEA) and DHEA-SULPHATE
3β
PROGESTERONE
17-α-OH-PROGESTERONE
ANDROSTENEDIONE
ESTRONE (E1)
21
11-DEOXYCORTICOSTERONE (DOC)
11-DEOXYCORTISOL (S)
TESTOSTERONE
ESTRADIOL-17β (E2)
ANDROGENS
ESTROGENS
11β
CORTICOSTERONE (B)
CORTISOL (HYDROCORTISONE, F)
GLUCOCORTICOIDS
18
18-OH-CORTICOSTERONE
ALDOSTERONE

4.27.) <u>OVARY</u> (Granulosa Cells)

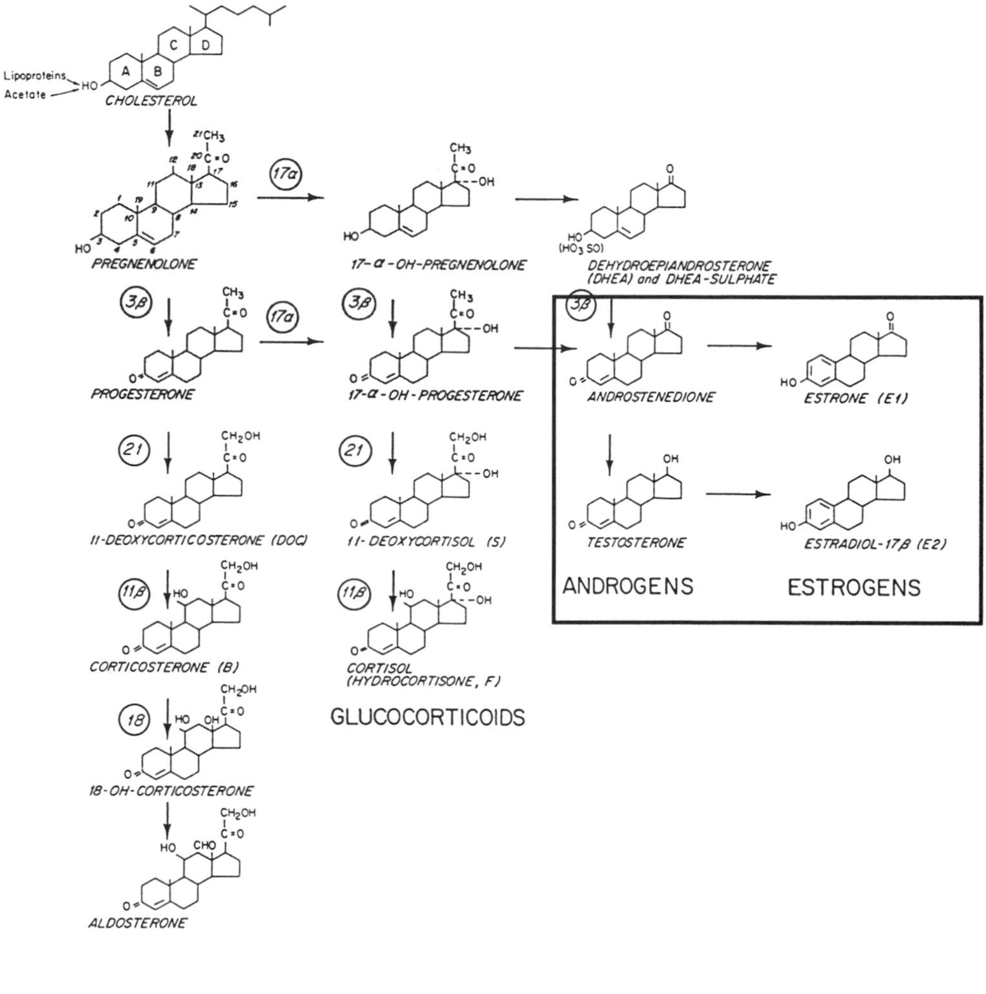

CHOLESTEROL

Lipoproteins
Acetate

PREGNENOLONE

17-α-OH-PREGNENOLONE

DEHYDROEPIANDROSTERONE
(DHEA) and DHEA-SULPHATE
(HO₃ SO)

PROGESTERONE

17-α-OH-PROGESTERONE

ANDROSTENEDIONE

ESTRONE (E1)

11-DEOXYCORTICOSTERONE (DOC)

11-DEOXYCORTISOL (S)

TESTOSTERONE

ESTRADIOL-17,β (E2)

ANDROGENS   ESTROGENS

CORTICOSTERONE (B)

CORTISOL
(HYDROCORTISONE, F)

GLUCOCORTICOIDS

18-OH-CORTICOSTERONE

ALDOSTERONE

4.28.) <u>PERIPHERAL METABOLISM</u>

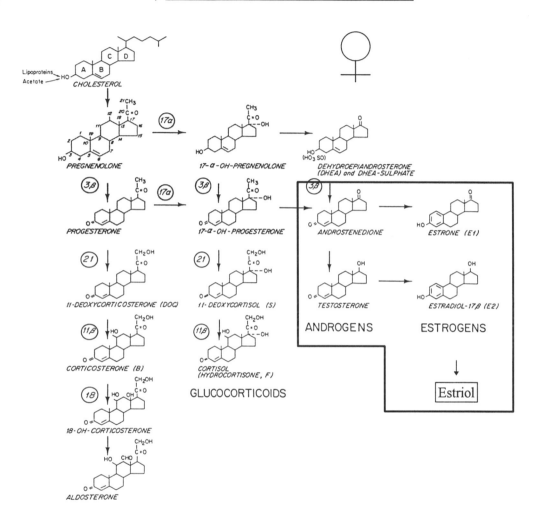

CHOLESTEROL

PREGNENOLONE

17-α-OH-PREGNENOLONE

DEHYDROEPIANDROSTERONE
(DHEA) and DHEA-SULPHATE

PROGESTERONE

17-α-OH-PROGESTERONE

ANDROSTENEDIONE

ESTRONE (E1)

11-DEOXYCORTICOSTERONE (DOC)

11-DEOXYCORTISOL (S)

TESTOSTERONE

ESTRADIOL-17β (E2)

CORTICOSTERONE (B)

CORTISOL
(HYDROCORTISONE, F)

ANDROGENS

ESTROGENS

18-OH-CORTICOSTERONE

GLUCOCORTICOIDS

Estriol

ALDOSTERONE

4.29.) <u>CORPUS LUTEUM</u>

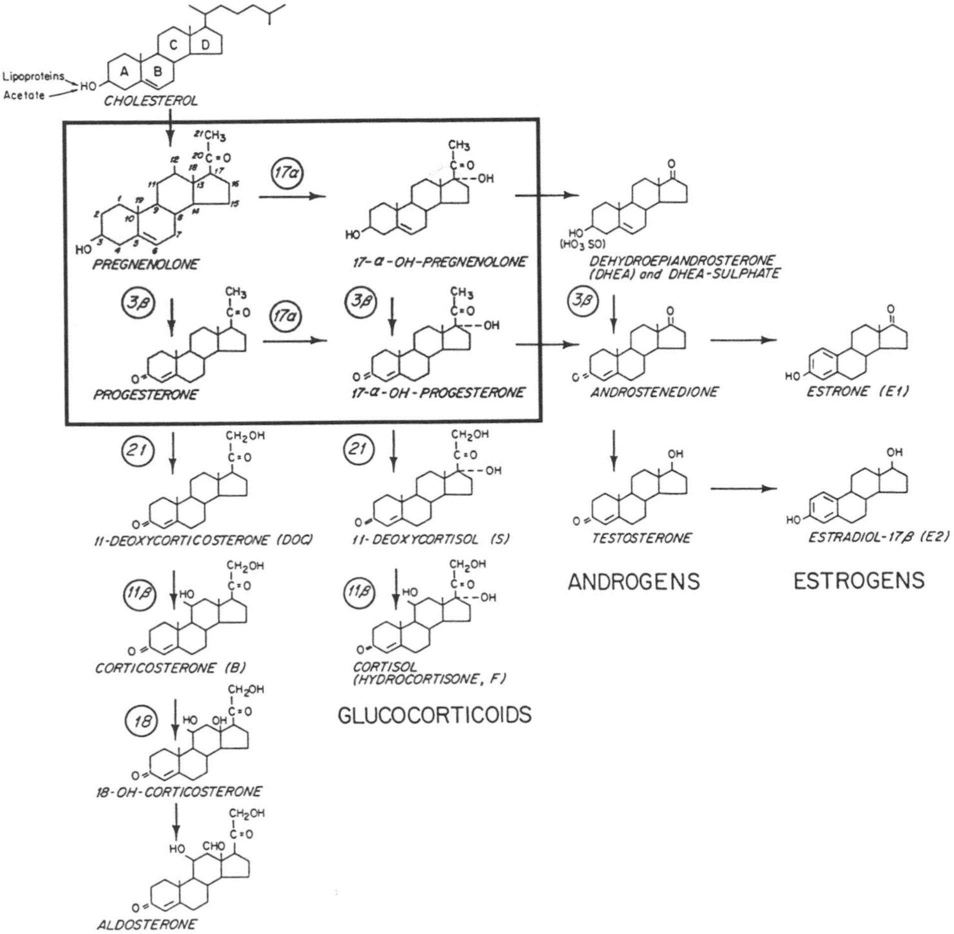

Lipoproteins
Acetate — CHOLESTEROL

PREGNENOLONE

(17α)

17-α-OH-PREGNENOLONE

DEHYDROEPIANDROSTERONE
(DHEA) and DHEA-SULPHATE

(3β) PROGESTERONE *(17α)* *(3β)* 17-α-OH-PROGESTERONE

(3β) ANDROSTENEDIONE

ESTRONE (E1)

(21) 11-DEOXYCORTICOSTERONE (DOC)

(21) 11-DEOXYCORTISOL (S)

TESTOSTERONE

ESTRADIOL-17β (E2)

(11β) CORTICOSTERONE (B)

(11β) CORTISOL
(HYDROCORTISONE, F)

ANDROGENS

ESTROGENS

GLUCOCORTICOIDS

(18) 18-OH-CORTICOSTERONE

ALDOSTERONE

4.30.) <u>17-α-HYDROXYLASE</u>

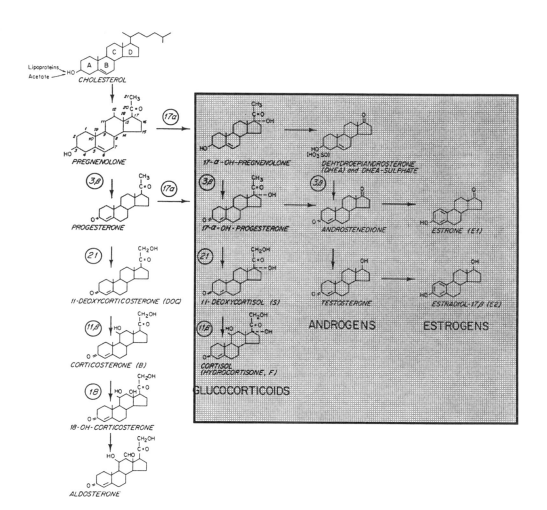

Male :   ambiguous genitalia
Female :   primary amenorrhea

4.31.) <u>21-α-HYDROXYLASE</u>

most common defect of
corticoid synthesis (95%)

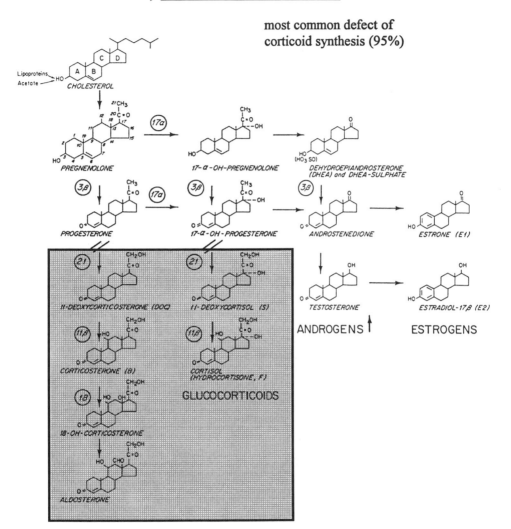

Male :   precocious puberty
Female :   ambiguous genitalia
saltwasting in 50-60% of patients

4.32.) <u>11-β-HYDROXYLASE</u>

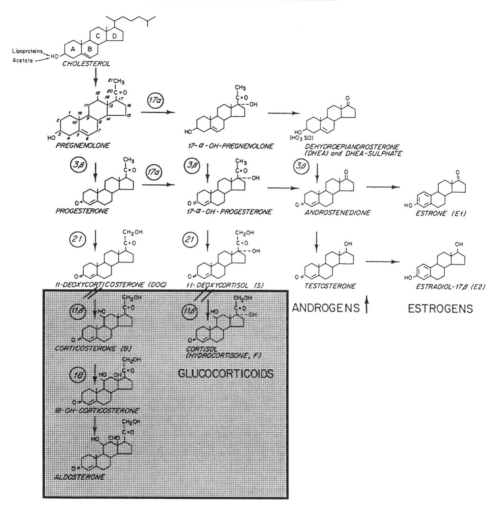

Male :   precocious puberty
Female :   ambiguous genitalia
hypertension, hypokalemia common

4.33.) <u>ENDOCRINE CONTROL OF METABOLISM</u>

	fat	sugar	proteins
insulin	A synthesis	A uptake (M,F) glycolysis (L,M) glycogen synthesis (L,M)	A synthesis
growth hormone	C lysis	C gluconeogenesis (L)	A synthesis
cortisol	C lysis redistribution	A inhibits uptake (M,F) gluconeogenesis (L) glycogen synthesis (L)	C degradation
epinephrine	C lysis	C increases uptake (M) glycolysis (M) gluconeogenesis (L) glycogenolysis (L,M)	-
glucagon	C lysis	C gluconeogenesis (L) glycogenolysis (L)	C increases uptake of AA in liver for gluconeogenesis

A: anabolic   **C: catabolic**

4.34.) <u>NUCLEOTIDES</u>

Base	Nucleoside	Nucleotide
adenine	adenosine	adenylate (AMP)
guanine	guanosine	guanylate (GMP)
uracil	uridine	uridylate (UMP)
cytosine	cytidine	cytidylate (CMP)
thymine	deoxythymidine	deoxythymidylate (dTMP)

4.35.) <u>PURINES</u>

<u>de novo</u>[1]

1.)   phosphoribosyl pyrophosphate --> IMP

2.)   IMP --> AMP or GMP

<u>salvage</u>[2]

hypoxanthine --> IMP   (*Lesch-Nyhan* !)

guanine   --> GMP

adenine   --> AMP

<u>degradation</u>

1.)   adenosine -> inosine -> hypoxanthine -> xanthine

guanosine -> guanine -> xanthine

2.)   xanthine -> uric Acid   (*allopurinol* !)

[1]**sugar first, then base**
[2]**base first, then sugar**

175

4.36.) PYRIMIDINES

de novo

1.)   glutamine --> carbamoylphosphate --> OMP --> UMP

2.)   UTP --> CTP

     dUMP --> dTMP

salvage

    uracil   --> UMP

    cytosine   --> CMP

degradation

ring can be opened and degraded --> acetyl CoA, succinyl CoA

4.37.) <u>REPLICATION</u>   DNA -> DNA

PROKARYOTE	EUKARYOTE
- helicase	- bidirectional, many forks
- primase	- α primer
- polymerase III	- δ, ε elongation
- 5' -> 3' polymerase	- β repair
- 3' exonuclease (proofreading)	- γ mitochondria
- 5' exonuclease (repair)	
- polymerase I	- no proofreading
- 5' -> 3' polymerase	- no exonuclease activity
- 5' exonuclease (removal of primer)	
- ligase	

4.38.) <u>INHIBITORS OF REPLICATION</u>

| anti-folates | **methotrexate** | - mammalian |
| | **trimethoprim** | - bacterial |
	pyrimethamine	- protozoal
purine analogs	**mercaptopurine**	- inhibits de novo synthesis
	azathioprine	- derivative of mercaptopurine
pyrimidine analogs	**cytarabine**	- ara-CTP, incorporated into DNA
	fluorouracil	- inhibits thymidylate synthesis
		(dUMP -> dTMP)
antibiotics	**actinomycin D**	- binds to DNA
	doxorubicin	- intercalates between base pairs
	bleomycin	- causes strand breaks in DNA

4.39.) <u>TRANSCRIPTION</u>   DNA -> RNA

PROKARYOTE	EUKARYOTE

- RNA polymerase
  holo enzyme : $\alpha_2\beta\beta'\ \sigma$
  core enzyme : $\alpha_2\beta\beta'$
	- polymerase I rRNA
	- polymerase II mRNA
	- polymerase III tRNA

- polycistronic mRNA	mRNA processing - cap : 7-methylguanosine triphosphate - tail : poly A - spliced by snRNA

4.40.) <u>INHIBITORS OF TRANSCRIPTION</u>

rifampicin	- binds to bacterial DNA-dependent RNA polymerase
	  inhibits initiation of RNA synthesis
	  anti-tuberculosis

α-amanitin	- blocks eukaryotic polymerase II mushroom poison

actinomycin D	- binds to DNA
	  inhibits transcription (low concentration)
	  inhibits replication (high concentration)

doxorubicin	- intercalates between base pairs inhibits translation and replication
streptodigin	- inhibits elongation of prokaryotic RNA synthesis

4.41.) <u>INHIBITORS OF TRANSLATION</u>
RNA -> Protein

<u>PROKARYOTES</u>

aminoglycosides	30 S	- inhibits initiation (binding of tRNA$_{fm}$)
tetracyclines	30 S	- inhibits binding of all other tRNAs
chloramphenicol	50 S	- inhibits peptidyl transferase
erythromycin	50 S	- inhibits translocation

<u>EUKARYOTES</u>

lectins	40/60 S	- inhibits initiation
cycloheximide	60 S	- inhibits peptidyl transferase
diphtheria toxin	60 S	- inhibits elongation factor

<u>PRO & EUKARYOTES</u>

puromycin		- incorporated into peptide chain premature chain termination

ANATOMY

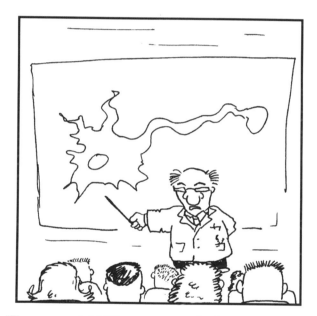

"There are 14 billion neurons in the brain and 14 billion *and one* facts to remember to pass the Boards."

5.1.) BRANCHIAL ARCHES

I	mandibular arch (Meckel)	malleus incus	muscles of mastication	facial artery	V3
II	hyoid arch (Reichert)	stapes styloid horns of hyoid	muscles of facial expression	ext. carotid artery	VII
III	thyrohyoid Arch	body of hyoid	stylopharyngeus	int. carotid artery	IX
IV	-	larynx	cricothyroid		X

PHARYNGEAL CLEFTS

I : (between Arch I and II)   ext. auditory meatus
II-IV :   cervical sinus (disappear or may form cervical cysts)

181

5.2.) <u>PHARYNGEAL POUCHES</u> [1]

I	tympanic cavity eustachian tube
II	palatine tonsil
III	ventral : thymus dorsal : <u>inf.</u> parathyroids
IV	ventral : - dorsal : <u>sup.</u> parathyroids
V	ultimobranchial body (parafollicular C cells)

[1] each corresponds to a pharyngeal cleft

5.3.) <u>FETAL REMNANTS</u>

umbilical artery	lat. umbilical ligament
umbilical vein	round ligament
ductus venosus	venous ligament
ductus arteriosus	ligamentum arteriosus
urachus	med. umbilical ligament
yolk stalk	Meckel's diverticle

5.4.) <u>UROGENITAL DEVELOPMENT</u>

	male	female
Müller[1]	disappears	- fallopian tubes - uterus - vagina down to hymen
Wolff[2]	- epididymis - vas deferens	disappears

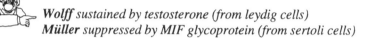

Wolff sustained by testosterone (from leydig cells)
Müller suppressed by MIF glycoprotein (from sertoli cells)

allantois	- urinary bladder - urachus
ureteric bud[3]	-trigonum - ureter - collecting tubules
pronephros	- disappears, never functional
mesonephros	- disappears, was functional
metanephros	- final kidney

[1] *also called paramesonephric duct*
[2] *also called mesonephric duct*
[3] *also called metanephric duct, (inf. part of mesonephric duct)*

5.5.) <u>**KEY DERMATOMES**</u>

skull	C2
thumb	C6
nipple	T5
belly button	T10
big toe	L4
penis	S3
anus	S5

knee jerk reflex	**L4**
ankle jerk reflex	**S1**

5.6.) <u>THE SKULL AND ITS HOLES</u>

optic	optic n. , ophthalmic a.
sup. orbital fissure	III, IV, V (ophthalm.), VI, sympath. nn., ophthalmic vv
rotundum	maxillary n.
ovale	mandibular n., access. meningeal a.
spinosum	middle meningeal a.
magnum	spinal cord, accessory n., vertebral aa., spinal aa.
jugular	IX, X, XI, pharyngeal a.
hypoglossal	XII, pharyngeal a.
int. aud. meatus	VII, VIII, labyrinthine a.

5.7.) <u>EYE</u>

med. rectus	nasal	III
lat. rectus	temporal	abducens VI
sup. rectus	up and nasal	III
sup. oblique	down and temporal	trochlear IV
inf. rectus	down and nasal	III
inf. oblique	up and temporal	III

dilator pupillae	mydriasis	sympathetic
sphincter pupillae	miosis	parasympathetic
ciliary	accommodation	parasympathetic

levator palpebrae sup.	ptosis	III
Müller's muscle	mild ptosis	sympathetic

5.8.) <u>MANDIBLE</u>

lat. pterygoid **digastric** **geniohyoid**	open mouth
masseter **med. pterygoid** **temporalis**	close mouth
lat. pterygoid	protrudes mandible
temporalis	retracts mandible
lat. pterygoid	lateral displacement

 these muscles are derived from the 1st branchial arch
-> innervated by mandibular nerve (V₃).

5.9.) <u>TONGUE</u>

A) MUSCLES

genioglossus	pulls it out
styloglossus	retracts it
hyoglossus	pulls it down

 - *All innervated by hypoglossus nerve (XII)*

- *If XII is damaged , tongue will deviate towards side of damage. (genioglossus of healthy side becomes dominant)*

B) SENSATION

	taste	touch, temperature
ant. 2/3 **post. 1/3**	VII IX	V3 IX

5.10.) **<u>LARYNX</u>**

A) MUSCLES

post. crico arytenoid	opens glottis	recurrent n.
lat. crico arytenoid	closes glottis	recurrent n.
crico thyroid	tightens vocal chords	sup. laryngeal n.
thyro arytenoid	relaxes vocal chords	recurrent n.

B) SENSATION

above glottis	sup. laryngeal nerve
below glottis	recurrent nerve

***left recurrent** nerve wraps around aortic arch.*
***right recurrent** nerve wraps around right subclavian artery.*

5.11.) <u>SHOULDER</u>

adduction	pectoralis major	C5-T1
abduction	first deltoid then serratus anterior	long thoracic n.
anteversion	deltoid	axillary n.
retroversion	teres major	
outward rotation	infraspinatus	
inward rotation	subscapular	

*"scapular winging" is due to damage to the long thoracic nerve.
(anterior serratus muscle)*

Rotator cuff :   **supraspinatus**
infraspinatus
teres minor
subscapularis

5.12.) __BRACHIAL PLEXUS__

upper trunk	C5-C6	musculocutaneous n. median n.
middle trunk	C7	axillary n. radial n.
lower trunk	C8-T1	median n. ulnar n.

	nerve injury
radial n.	- wrist drop - loss of triceps reflex
median n.	- no flexion of thumb, index and middle finger - no thumb opposition - thenar atrophy
ulnar n.	- claw hand - no flexion of 4th and 5th finger - apothenar atrophy
musculocutaneous n.	- no elbow flexion - no supination - loss of biceps reflex

5.13.) <u>ELBOW</u>

flexion	biceps brachii	musculocutaneous n.
extension	triceps brachii	radial n.
supination	biceps brachii	musculocutaneous n.
pronation	pronator teres	median n.

 "tennis elbow" is due to inflammation of the lateral epicondyle, which is the origin of extensor muscles ("backhand").

5.14.) <u>HIP</u>

outward rotation	gluteus maximus	inf. gluteal n.
inward rotation	gluteus medius et minimus	sup. glut. n.
extension	gluteus maximus	inf. gluteal n.
flexion	iliopsoas	femoral n.
abduction	gluteus medius	sup. gluteal n.
adduction	adductor magnus et minimus	obturator n.

 in femur neck fracture, the leg is abduced and externally rotated.

5.15.) <u>KNEE</u>

extension	quadriceps femoris	femoral n.
flexion	"hamstrings" - semimembranous muscle - semitendinous muscle - biceps femoris	sciatic n.
inward rotation	semimembranous	sciatic n.
outward rotation	biceps femoris	sciatic n.

 Sciatic nerve divides into tibial nerve and common peroneal nerve.

5.16.) <u>ANKLE</u>

	invert	evert
dorsiflex	tibialis anterior[1]	peroneus tertius[2]
plantarflex	tibialis posterior[3]	peroneus longus et brevis[4]

[1] deep peroneal nerve
[2] deep peroneal nerve
[3] tibial nerve
[4] superficial peroneal nerve

 Injury to common peroneal n. results in inability to dorsiflex
Injury to tibial nerve results in inability to invert foot.

Deep peroneal nerve innervates skin between 1st and 2nd toe.

5.17.) __HEART__

left coronary artery
  - ant. interventricular[1]
  - circumflex
	left ventricle
	septum
	AV node

right coronary artery	right ventricle sinus node

[1] most common occlusion.

5.18.) __PERITONEUM__

intraperitoneal	retroperitoneal
stomach small bowel transverse colon spleen (liver)	aorta vena cava kidneys pancreas duodenum ascending colon descending colon

5.19.) <u>ABDOMINAL ARTERIES</u>

celiac trunk	stomach spleen liver duodenum	left gastric art. splenic art. hepatic art. gastroduodenal art. sup. pancreaticoduodenal art.
sup. mesenteric art.	duodenum small intestine cecum ascending colon transverse colon	inf. pancreaticoduodenal art. > many branches
inf. mesenteric art.	descending colon sigmoid rectum	> many branches sup. rectal art.

ovary	aorta -> ovarian artery internal iliac a. -> uterine artery
testes	aorta -> testicular artery internal iliac a. -> art. of ductus deferens inf. epigastric a. -> cremasteric artery

5.20.) <u>LAYERS OF SPERMATIC CORD</u>

loose connective tissue	arteries, pampiniform plexus
internal spermatic fascia	from fascia transversalis
cremaster muscle and fascia	from int. oblique muscle
external spermatic fascia	from ext. oblique aponeurosis
superficial fascia	contains dartos muscle

5.21.) <u>CORTEX</u>

vision	occipital lobe
hearing	temporal lobe
taste	insula, below postcentral gyrus
reading, writing	angular gyrus
primary motor cortex	precentral
primary sensory cortex	postcentral
Wernicke (sensory)	temporal lobe, upper gyrus
Broca (motor)	frontal lobe, at lateral fissure

5.22.) <u>BRAIN ARTERIES</u>

ophthalmic a.	unilateral blindness
post. cerebral a.	homonymous hemianopsia
middle cerebral a.	lateral cortex (motor & sensory, upper body)
ant. cerebral a.	medial cortex (motor & sensory, legs and feet)
ant. choroidal a.	internal capsule
cerebellar arteries	ataxia brainstem syndromes

5.23.) <u>CRANIAL NERVES</u>

somatic motor	III	extraocular eye muscles (except sup.obl. and lat. rect.)
	IV	superior oblique
	VI	lateral rectus
	XII	tongue muscles (except palatoglossus)
branchial motor[1]	V	mastication
	VII	facial expression
	IX, X	pharynx, larynx
	XI	trapezius, sternocleidomastoid muscles
visceral motor	III	ciliary muscle, constrictor pupillae
	VII	all glands except parotid
	IX	parotid
	X	abdominal viscera up to splenic flexure
special sensory	I	smell
	II	vision
	VII, IX	taste
	VIII	hearing, balance
general sensory	V, VII, IX, X	pain, temperature, touch, proprioception
visceral sensory	IX, X	afferents for visceral reflexes

[1] innervate skeletal muscle derived from branchial arches

5.24.) __PARASYMPATHETIC GANGLIA__

Nucleus	Nerve	Ganglion	Structure
Edinger-Westphal	III	ciliary	eye
sup. salivary nucl.	VII	sublingual submaxillary	lacrimal gland nasal glands submandibular gland
inf. salivary nucl.	IX	otic	parotid gland
dorsal motor nucl.	X	many, mostly intramural	many

5.25.) <u>BASAL GANGLIA</u>

striatum	caudate putamen globus pallidum
neostriatum	caudate putamen
paleostriatum	globus pallidum
lentiform nucleus	putamen globus pallidum

5.26.) <u>THALAMUS</u>

med. thalamus	amygdala prefrontal cortex
lat. thalamus	pulvinar output to cortex
ventral anterior nucl.	basal ganglia
ventral posterior nucl.	**VPL** : med. lemniscus proprioception, touch etc. **VPM** : nerve V , taste
ventro lateral	input from cerebellum
post. thalamic nucl.	**med.** geniculate : **acoustic** **lat.** geniculate : **optical**
ant. thalamus (limbic system)	input : mammillary bodies output : cingula

5.27.) MEDULLA

lateral :

post. inf. cerebellar art.

spinothalamic tract
ncl. solitarius
ncl. ambiguus

spinal tract nucl. V

reticular formation

"WALLENBERG"

- contralat. pain/temp loss on body
- ipsilat. loss of taste
- hoarseness
- loss of pharyngeal reflex
- ipsilateral pain/temp loss on face

- ipsilateral Horner's

medial :

ant. spinal art.

med. lemniscus

hypoglossal muscle
pyramidal tract

- contralat. loss of position sense
- contralat. loss of vibration sense
- ipsilat. hemiparesis of tongue
- contralat. hemiparesis

5.28.) <u>LOWER PONS</u>

lateral :

ant. inf. cerebellar art.

spinocerebellar tract	- ipsilat. limb ataxia
spinal tract nucl. V	- ipsilat. loss of cutaneous sensation from face
nucleus VII	- ipsilat. paralysis upper&lower face
vestibular nucl.	- vertigo
cochlear nuclei	- nerve deafness
reticular formation	- ipsilateral Horner's

medial :

basilar artery

corticospinal tract	- contralat. hemiparesis
med. lemniscus	- contralat. loss of position and vibration sense
med. long. fasciculus	- ipsilat. eye can not adduct on lateral gaze
nucl. VI	- ipsilat. paralysis of lat. rectus oculi
nucl VII	- ipsilat. facial paralysis

5.29.) <u>UPPER PONS</u>

lateral :

sup. cerebellar art.

spinothalamic tract	- contralat. loss of pain sensation from body
motor nucl. V	- ipsilat. loss of masseter function
reticular formation	- ipsilateral Horner's

medial :

basilar art.

corticospinal tract	contralat. hemiparesis

208

PHYSIOLOGY

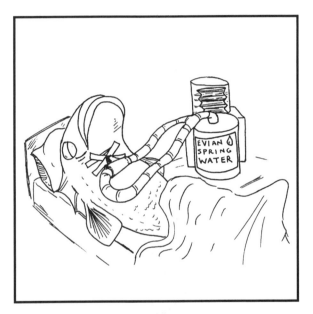

Fish respirators.

6.1.) <u>SIX EQUATIONS YOU REALLY NEED</u>

<u>HEART</u>

Blood pressure

$$P_{average} = P_{diastolic} + 1/3 \, (P_{systolic} - P_{diastolic})$$

Fick's Principle

cardiac output = oxygen uptake / (a-v oxygen difference)

<u>KIDNEY</u>

Clearance of X

$$clearance \cdot [X]_{plasma} = urine \; flow \cdot [X]_{urine}$$

<u>LUNG</u>

Diffusion (Fick)

$$flux = D \cdot area \cdot \frac{concentration \; gradient}{membrane \; thickness}$$

Elasticity

$$elasticity = \frac{\Delta \; pressure}{\Delta \; volume}$$

$$compliance = 1/elasticity = \frac{\Delta \; volume}{\Delta \; pressure}$$

<u>BLOOD</u>

Henderson-Hasselbach

$$pH = pK + \log \frac{[salt]}{[acid]}$$

$$pH = pK + \log \frac{[HCO_3^-]}{[CO_2]}$$

note: H_2CO_3 is in equilibrium with CO_2
kidneys regulate HCO_3^-
lung regulates CO_2 (i.e. H_2CO_3)

6.2.) <u>ION CHANNELS</u>

K$^+$	- resting membrane potential (RMP) - repolarization
Na$^+$	- action potential - rapid inactivation (refractory period)
Ca^{2+}	- excitation contraction coupling - excitation secretion coupling - cardiac pacemaker (sinus node, AV node) - cardiac plateau phase - ryanodine receptor
cations	- depolarization - dark current of photoreceptors - motor endplate
Cl$^-$	- CNS, postsynaptic potentials
Na$^+$ / K$^+$ pump	- maintains ion gradients - direct contribution to RMP is small !

6.3.) <u>SIGNAL TRANSDUCTION</u>

α1, M1, H1 **angiotensin II** **tachykinins** **endothelin**	IP3, DAG
β, H2 **ACTH**	cAMP increase
α2 **M2, M3**	cAMP decrease
EDRF (NO) **ANP**	cGMP
insulin **growth factors**	tyrosine kinase
steroid hormones **thyroid hormones** **retinoic acid**	gene expression

6.4.) <u>EEG</u>

awake attentive awake relaxed	**beta** >12 / min **alpha** 8-12 / min
sleep I	**theta** 4-8 / min
sleep II	low voltage / spindles
sleep III/IV	**delta** 1-4 / min
REM	beta & theta

6.5.) <u>SLEEP</u>

REM	Non REM
erections in males	enuresis (first half of night)
total muscle relaxation (except, fingers, toes, eyes)	somnambulism
dreams, nightmares	night terrors

6.6.) EPILEPSY

grand mal	- tonic, then clonic - loss of consciousness - incontinence - EEG : high voltage spikes
petit mal	- absence seizure ("blank spell") - no loss of muscle tone - EEG : 3/sec spikes and domes
narcolepsy	- loss of muscle tone - REM onset sleep
psychomotor	- non-goal directed activity (lip smacking, walking...) - EEG : spikes in temporal lobes
Jacksonian	- spreading muscle group activity (e.g. fingers -> forearm -> shoulder) - EEG : focal around antral sulcus

6.7.) <u>NERVES</u>

Aα [1]	- efferent : sk. muscle - afferent : from muscle spindle
Aγ	- efferent : to muscle spindle
Aβ , Aδ	- afferent : touch, fast pain
C	- afferent : slow pain
B , C [2]	- efferent : autonomic nerves

[1] *diameter large, conduction velocity high*
[2] *diameter small, conduction velocity low*

6.8.) <u>TOUCH</u>

pressure	Merkel [1]
touch	Meissner hair follicles
vibration	Pacini [2]

[1] *slowly adapting*
[2] *rapidly adapting*

6.9.) <u>ACCOMMODATION</u>

close	far
ciliary muscle contracted	ciliary muscle relaxed
zonula fibers relaxed	zonula fibers tense
lens rounded (if elastic)	lens flat
focal length short	focal length far

myopia (nearsightedness)	- lens has normal elasticity - focal point too short (or eye ball too long) - corrected with negative lens
hypermetropia [1] (farsightedness)	- lens has normal elasticity - focal point too far (or eye ball too short) - corrected with positive lens - often confused with presbyopia
presbyopia [1] (age)	- lens has lost elasticity - cannot shorten focal length - corrected with positive lens

[1] difficulty reading

6.10.) <u>NYSTAGMUS</u>

optokinetic	- looking out of train *against movement of image*
vestibular	- postrotational *against direction of prior rotation* - temperature *away from cold ear*

 direction of nystagmus defined by <u>fast</u> phase.

6.11.) <u>COCHLEA</u>

scala vestibuli	Na⁺ rich	perilymph
scala media	K⁺ rich	endolymph
scala tympani	Na⁺ rich	perilymph

 basilar membrane between media and tympani.
endocochlear potential : Scala media = +80 mV

6.12.) <u>TUNING FORK</u>

	Weber	Rinne
method	place fork on top of skull	place fork on mastoid process until tone disappears. Then hold next to ear.
conduction deafness (middle ear)	sound lateralized to sick ear	bone conduction better than air conduction
nerve deafness (inner ear)	sound lateralized to normal ear	air conduction better than bone conduction

6.13.) <u>AUTONOMIC NERVOUS SYSTEM</u>

	sympathetic	parasympathetic
heart	increased heart rate increased conduction increased force	decreased heart rate
bronchi	dilates	constricts
GI tract	reduces motility	increases motility
sphincters of GI tract	constricts	relaxes
rectum	allows filling	empties relaxes internal sphincter
bladder	allows filling	empties relaxes internal sphincter
erection		maintains erection
ejaculation	triggers ejaculation	
pupils of eye	big (mydriasis)	small (miosis)
sweat glands	sweat (cholinergic !)	
salivary glands		secretion
blood vessels	depends on receptors: - α constricts - β dilates	no direct effect (except artery of penis)

6.14.) __RECEPTORS__

nicotinic	**- autonomic ganglia** both sympathetic and parasympathetic ! - adrenal medulla **- neuromuscular junction** these differ from autonomic ones !
muscarinic	**- postsynaptic parasympathetic** **- sweat glands** (innervated by sympathetic nerves)
alpha 1	**- postsynaptic sympathetic** generally excitatory (vasoconstriction) in GI tract inhibitory
alpha 2	**- presynaptic sympathetic** (decrease catecholamine release) **- central nervous system** (decrease sympathetic tone)
beta 1	**- postsynaptic sympathetic (cardiac)** excitatory (chronotrop, dromotrop, inotrop)
beta 2	**- postsynaptic sympathetic (all others)** inhibitory (vasodilation, bronchodilation)

 Four ways to decrease blood pressure :

1. block nicotinic ganglionic receptors
2. block β receptors
3. block α1 receptors
4. stimulate α2 receptors

6.15.) <u>CONTROL OF HEART BEAT</u>

right vagus nerve	- slows frequency (sinus node)

left vagus nerve	- slows conduction
	  (AV node)
	
	- decreased force of contraction
	  (atria but not ventricles !)

sympathetic	- increased frequency - increased conduction - increased force of contraction (atria and ventricles)
epinephrine	- increased conduction & contraction - increased frequency
norepinephrine	- increased conduction & contraction - decreased frequency (baroreceptor reflex !)

6.16.) <u>CONTROL OF MUSCLE TONE</u>

muscle spindle	- muscle length - activates α motoneuron	γ efferent 1A afferent
Golgi	- muscle tension - inhibits α motoneuron	1B afferent

<u>increased muscle tone</u> :
activation of γ fibers
upper motor neuron lesions (hemiplegia)
Parkinson
cold, anxiety

<u>decreased muscle tone</u> :
lower motor neuron lesions
spinal shock (early phase of hemiplegia)
warm

6.17.) <u>MUSCLE TYPES</u>

	red muscle	white muscle
myosin isoenzyme	slow	fast
glycolytic capacity	low	high
oxidative capacity	high	low

oxidative capacity

 <u>related to</u>
 - number of capillaries
 - myoglobin content
 - number of mitochondria

6.18.) <u>ELECTROMECHANICAL COUPLING</u>

sk. muscle	heart muscle	smooth muscle
motor units	syncytium	syncytium
AP 2-4 ms	AP 200-400 ms	- tonic - phasic (slow waves, spikes)
troponin	troponin	calmodulin MLC phosphorylation
Ca^{2+} from SR	Ca^{2+} influx	Ca^{2+} influx / SR
tetanus	no tetanus	myogenic tone

6.19.) <u>REGULATION OF FORCE</u>

sk. muscle	heart muscle	smooth muscle
- recruitment of motor units - AP frequency	- AP duration	- membrane potential - biochemical modifications

6.20.) __BLOOD__

serum = plasma - fibrinogen

pre-albumin	- thyroxine, Vit.A
albumin	- oncotic pressure - binds hormones, drugs etc.
α1 globulin	- lipoproteins - α1 antitrypsin
α2 globulin	- haptoglobin (carries hemoglobin dimers)
β globulin	- transferrin (carries iron)
γ globulin	- antibodies

6.21.) <u>BLOOD CELLS</u>

erythrocytosis	- lack of oxygen - kidney tumors (erythropoetin)
leukocytosis	- infections - leukemia
leukopenia	- radiation - cytostatic drugs
thrombocytopenia	- DIC - idiopathic

6.22.) <u>CYTOKINES</u>

	produced by	action
α-interferon	leukocytes	antiviral induces MHC-I
β-interferon	fibroblasts	antiviral
γ-interferon	T cells	activates macrophages induces MHC-II
TNF	macrophages	fever, cachexis etc.
IL-1	macrophages	fever
IL-2, IL-3, IL-4, IL-5	T cells	activate many other cells
IL-6	macrophages fibroblasts	activates B cells
IL-7	bone marrow cells	proliferation of B and T cells
PDGF	platelets endothelial cells	proliferation of vascular smooth muscle cells

6.23.) <u>HEMOGLOBINS</u>

embryonal	Gower 1	$\zeta_2\varepsilon_2$
fetal	HbF	$\alpha_2\gamma_2$
adult	HbA HbA_2 HbA_{1C}	$\alpha_2\beta_2$ (98%) $\alpha_2\delta_2$ (2%) glycosylated derivative
sickle cells	HbS	$\alpha_2\beta^s_2$
α-thalassemia	HbH Hb Bart	β_4 γ_4
β-thalassemia		$\alpha_2\gamma_2$ $\alpha_2\delta_2$

6.24.) <u>OXYGEN BINDING CURVE</u>

right shift	**= reduced binding of O$_2$** increased protons (low pH) increased CO$_2$ increased 2,3-DPG increased temperature
left shift	**= tighter binding of O$_2$** fetal hemoglobin myoglobin

	arterial	venous
PO$_2$	95 mmHg	40 mmHg
O$_2$ saturation	97 %	70 %
PCO$_2$	40 mmHg	45 mm Hg
pH	7.4	7.37

6.25.) <u>CIRCULATION</u>

perfusion (rest) (in % of cardiac output)	kidney > brain, muscle > heart
perfusion (exercise) (in % of cardiac output)	muscle >> heart > brain > kidney
specific perfusion (rest) (in ml min^{-1} / g tissue)	kidney >> heart > brain > muscle
largest pressure	arteries
largest resistance	arterioles
largest cross-sectional area	capillaries
largest volume	veins

 <u>orthostasis (standing up)</u> :
systolic pressure unchanged
diastolic pressure increased
peripheral resistance increased
heart rate increased

6.26.) FETAL CIRCULATION

foramen ovale	right atrium -> left atrium
ductus arteriosus	pulmonary artery -> aorta
ductus venosus	umbilical vein -> vena cava inf.

Ductus arteriosus kept open by prostaglandins.
Lung maturation accelerated by glucocorticoids.

Placenta receives 30-40% of fetal blood circulation.

Head and upper extremities (preductal) receive O_2 rich blood.
Lower extremities (postductal) receive mixed blood.

6.27.) <u>CARDIAC CYCLE</u>

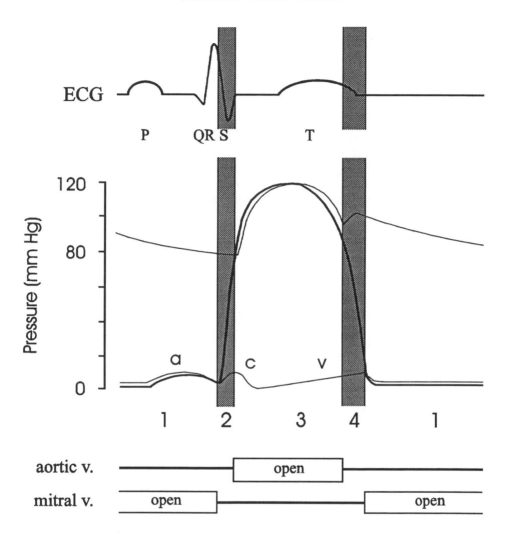

ECG

P   QR S   T

Pressure (mm Hg)

120

80

a   c   v

0

1   2   3   4   1

aortic v. —————————— open ——————————

mitral v. ———— open ———— open

1 - filling   **a-wave** : atrial contraction
2 - isovolumetric contraction   **c-wave** : bulging of mitral valve
3 - ejection   **v-wave** : filling of atria
4 - isovolumetric relaxation

233

6.28.) <u>LUNG VOLUMES</u>

IRV = 3.0 ⎫
          ⎬   IC = 3.5 ⎫
IV = 0.5 ⎭   ⎬   VC = 4.7 ⎫
                       ⎭   ⎬
ERV = 1.2 ⎫   ⎬   TC = 6.0
          ⎬   FRC = 2.5 ⎭   ⎭
RV = 1.3 ⎭

IRV, IV and ERV measured by spirometer
RV measured by helium dilution

Ventilation = dV/dt

alveolar ventilation = ventilation - deadspace ventilation

dead space = anatomical plus unperfused alveoli

dead space measured by nitrogen exhalation
(inhale 100% oxygen, measure N_2 while exhaling)

Ventilation / Perfusion ratio V/Q

V is higher at **base** of lung than at tip
Q is higher at **base** of lung than at tip
V/Q is higher at **tip** of lung than at base !

(that's why tubercle bacilli are found at tips of lung,
while pneumonia tends to develop at base of lungs)

6.29.) <u>BREATHING PATTERNS</u>

Cheyne-Stokes	**- waxing and waning** - uremia - can be physiological at high altitude
Kussmaul	**- deep inspirations** - compensation of metabolic acidosis (e.g. diabetic ketoacidosis)
Biot	**- apneic episodes** - brain tumors

Sleep apnea can be a) central (decreased responsiveness to CO_2)
b) obstructive (tongue falls back)

Chronic lung insufficiency
-> central CO_2 receptors become less responsive
-> peripheral O_2 receptors become "more important"
-> do not administer pure O_2 (or patient may stop breathing!)

6.30.) <u>RESPIRATORY QUOTIENT</u>
(CO_2 release / O_2 uptake)

	kcal / g	RQ
carbohydrates	4	1.0
proteins	4	0.8
fat	9	0.7

RQ < 0.7	- hypoventilation - diabetes - fasting
RQ > 1.0	- hyperventilation

6.31.) ACID BASE

	pH	primary disturbance	compensatory response	
respiratory acidosis	< 7.35	PCO_2 ↑	HCO_3^- ↑	- lung edema etc. - central (brain tumor)
metabolic acidosis	< 7.35	HCO_3^- ↓	PCO_2 ↓	- diabetes (ketoacidosis) - shock (lactate) - diarrhea
respiratory alkalosis	> 7.45	PCO_2 ↓	HCO_3^- ↓	- high altitude - anxiety
metabolic alkalosis	> 7.45	HCO_3^- ↑	PCO_2 ↑	- vomiting - diuretics

6.32.) <u>TRANSPORT</u>

	passive	facilitated	active
energy (ATP)	no	no	yes
against gradient	no	no	yes
specific	no	yes	yes
saturating	no	yes	yes

6.33.) <u>RENAL TRANSPORT</u>

prox. tubule	- active resorption
	  (glucose, amino acids etc.)
	
	- active secretion
	  (organic acids, protons etc.)
	
	- carbonic anhydrase inhibitors

Henle loop	- NaCl resorption - water impermeable ! (generates osmotic gradient) *- loop diuretics*
dist. tubule	- K^+ secretion, H^+ secretion (in exchange for Na^+) *- thiazide diuretics*
collecting duct	- water permeable (depending on ADH)

<u>Titratable acids</u> :
H^+ (<1%), uric acid (10%), phosphate (40%)
<u>Non-titratable acids</u> :
NH_4^+ (50%)

6.34.) <u>CLEARANCE</u>

	value	calculated from measurement of...
RBF (renal blood flow)	1200 ml / min	PAH clearance hematocrit
RPF (renal plasma flow)	600 ml / min	PAH clearance
GFR (glomerular filtration rate)	125 ml / min	inulin clearance or creatinin clearance
FF (filtration fraction)	20 %	GFR / RPF

clearance > GFR	filtration + net secretion
clearance = GFR	filtration only (or secretion = resorption)
clearance < GFR	filtration + net resorption

contraction of afferent arteriole decreases GFR.
contraction of efferent arteriole increases GFR.

6.35.) <u>VOLUME REGULATION</u>

	receptors	effect
osmo regulation	hypothalamus	thirst ADH release
volume regulation	baroreceptors	sympathetic activation renin -> ang. II -> aldosterone

	ICV	ECV	
hypotone dehydration	↑	↓	- diarrhea, vomiting
isotone dehydration	∅	↓	- blood loss
hypertone dehydration	↓	↓	- excessive sweating - diabetes insipidus
hypotone hydration	↑	↑	- SIADH
isotone hydration	∅	↑	- cardiac failure - nephrotic syndrome
hypertone hydration	↓	↑	- hyperaldosteronism

6.36.) RENIN ET Al.

angiotensinogen	liver	α2 globulin
(renin)	kidney (JGA)	protease
angiotensin I		
(converting enzyme)	lung	protease
angiotensin II		vasoconstriction
aldosterone	z. glomerulosa	Na$^+$reabsorption K$^+$ secretion
atrial natriuretic peptide (ANP)	when atria are stretched (high ECV)	natriuresis
natriuretic factor	ouabain-like inhibitor of Na$^+$/K$^+$ pump	unknown significance

JG cells are epitheloid cells of afferent arteriole
macula densa is modified epithelium of distal tubule juxtaglomerular.

Renin is released when : blood pressure is low at JG cells.
 NaCl delivery to macula densa is low.

Patients with Bartter's syndrome :
 high renin, Ang II and aldosterone, but normotensive!
 (down regulation of vascular Ang.II receptors ?)

Patients with hypertension respond to ACE inhibitors even when their
 renin levels are normal or low!

6.37.) <u>INTESTINAL ABSORPTION</u>

sugars	ileum	jejunum
amino acids [1]	ileum	jejunum
iron	duodenum	
vit. B12		**terminal ileum**
bile salts		**terminal ileum**

<u>Iron</u> :
absorbed as Fe $^{2+}$ (combine with anti-oxidants, e.g. Vit.C)
transported as transferrin
stored as ferritin and hemosiderin

[1] *<u>specific transporters</u>*
Hartnup disease *: defect in neutral aminoacid transporter*
cystinuria : *defect in basic aminoacid transporter*

6.38.) STOMACH

chief cells	- pepsinogen
parietal cells	- HCl - intrinsic factor
G cells (antrum)	- gastrin

6.39.) GI HORMONES

	released by...	results in...
gastrin	- vagus (ACh) - peptides, alcohol and alkaline pH in stomach	- increased stomach motility - delayed stomach emptying - HCl secretion
secretin	- fat, acids and peptides in duodenum	- HCO_3^- rich pancreatic secretion - gallbladder secretions
CCK	- fat, acids and peptides in duodenum	- enzyme rich pancreatic secretion - gallbladder contractions
GIP	- glucose, fat in duodenum	- stimulates insulin secretion
somatostatin	- acid in stomach	- inhibits G cells

6.40.) ADRENAL HORMONES

	released by...	pathology
aldosterone	basal secretion ! Ang II high K$^+$ (ACTH)	<u>**Conn**</u> (hyper...) - K$^+$ depletion - hypertension - but not edematous ! - not hypernatremic ! - weakness, tetany <u>**Addison**</u> (hypo...) - Na$^+$ loss (hypotension) - K$^+$ retention - H$^+$ retention (met. acidosis) - pigmentation
glucocorticoids	stress ACTH	<u>**Cushing**</u> (hyper...) - skin atrophy - muscle wasting - moon face - decreased glucose tolerance - poor wound healing - osteoporosis

Most adrenalectomized patients could survive on mineralcorticoids alone, but would face potentially fatal hypoglycemic episodes.

6.41.) GONADOTROPE HORMONES

	ovary	testes
FSH	follicle maturation	spermatogenesis
LH = ICSH	triggers ovulation luteinization of follicle	testosterone secretion (Leydig cells)

6.42.) <u>GENE EXPRESSION</u>

operon	promoter + operator + structural genes
repressor	- protein that binds to DNA (operator) and prevents transcription. - metabolite (e.g. lactose) binds to repressor and prevents its interaction with DNA
regulator gene	- codes for repressor
TATA factor	- transcription factor (protein) - binds to TATAAA box (part of promoter) - eukaryotic RNA polymerase cannot recognize promoter in absence of transcription factor !
enhancer	- regulatory DNA sequence - can be upstream or downstream of promoter

SOCIAL SCIENCE

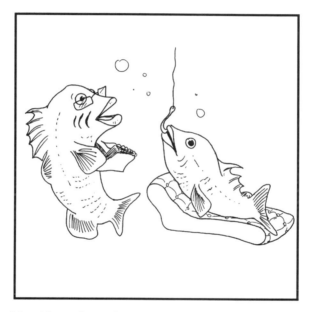

"And how long have you been feeling that
people are after you?"

7.1.) <u>CANCER EPIDEMIOLOGY</u>

A.) <u>Incidence</u>

male	female
1. lung	1. breast
2. prostate	2. colon
3. colon	3. lung

B.) <u>Mortality</u>

male	female
1. lung	1. lung
2. colon	2. breast
3. prostate	3. colon

 Prevalence depends on a) incidence, b) duration of disease.

7.2.) <u>MOTOR DEVELOPMENT</u>

chin up	1 month
chest up	2 month
knee push and "swim"	6 month
sits alone / stands with help	7 month
crawls on stomach	8 month
stands holding on furniture	10 month
walks when led	11 month
stands alone	14 month
walks alone	15 month

7.3.) PSYCHOLOGICAL DEVELOPMENT

years	Erikson	Freud	Piaget
0 - 1.5	trust / mistrust	ORAL (trust & dependence)	senso-motoric
1.5 - 3	autonomy / shame	ANAL (holding vs. letting out)	pre-operational
3 - 6	initiative / guilt	PHALLIC (Oedipus complex)	concrete operational
6 - 13	industry / inferiority	LATENCY	formal operational
13 - 18	identity / role confusion	GENITAL	
18 - 25	intimacy / isolation		
25 - 50	generativity / stagnation		
50 - ?	integrity / despair		

7.4.) <u>IQ TESTS</u>

Deviation Tests	**Tests of Mental Age**
mean : 100 **standard dev. : 15** normed for each age group	IQ = mental age / biological age
WAIS adults **WISC** children **WPPSI** preschool	**Stanford Binet** (for children 3-12 yrs.)

<u>Degrees of Mental Retardation</u>

IQ 55 - 70 (mild)	mentally handicapped educatable
IQ 40 - 55 (moderate)	trainable for personal hygiene
IQ 25 - 40 (severe)	custodial
IQ < 25 (profound)	custodial

7.5.) <u>CONDITIONING</u>

"classic"	"operant"
unconditioned stimulus : meat **unconditioned response** : salivation	**operant** : behavior to be modified
conditioned stimulus : bell **conditioned response** : salivation	**pos. reinforcer** : candy **neg. reinforcer** : shock **primary reward** : food, sex **secondary reward** : money, praise
works on reflexive behavior (autonomic nervous system)	works on autonomic nervous system or complex behavior
reinforcement (UCS) occurs regardless of response.	reward (or punishment) depends on response
partial reinforcement hastens extinction.	partial reinforcement results in greater resistance to extinction. (e.g. gambling addiction)

7.6.) <u>PSYCHOPATHOLOGY</u>

schizophrenia	- defect in reality testing - affect incongruence - ambivalence - associations - autism - auditory hallucinations
delirium	- acute onset - fluctuating consciousness - disorientation - optical hallucinations
dementia	- slow onset - no impairment of consciousness - loss of intellectual functions
neurosis	- phobic neurosis - anxiety neurosis - obsessive compulsive n. - hysterical neurosis - patients are distressed knowing that their symptoms are irrational
personality disorders	- narcistic, dependent, paranoid, schizoid, antisocial - borderline[1] - patients are not distressed, spouses and public suffer

[1] has both neurotic and psychotic components

7.7.) <u>SOMATOFORM DISORDERS</u>

somatization (Briquet's syndrome)	- sickly for most of life - GI, reproductive, cardiopulmonary, pain etc. - diagnosed, when at least 12 symptoms are present and history of several years.
conversion disorder (hysterical neurosis)	- "pseudoneurological" blindness, paresthesia, paralysis - symptoms begin and end suddenly - often misdiagnosed as "malingering"
hypochondriasis	- unrealistic interpretation of body signs - belief to have serious disease that goes unrecognized by family and physicians

7.8.) <u>SENSITIVITY / SPECIFICITY</u>

	patient is sick	patient is healthy
test result is positive	A	B
test result is negative	C	D

Sensitivity : divide A by (A+C)

Definition :   Sensitivity is the probability that a sick patient (A+C) will have a positive test result (A).

Example :   A test has a sensitivity of 90% means that 10% of patients with the disease go undetected (C = false negative) !

	patient is sick	patient is healthy
test result is positive	A	B
test result is negative	C	D

Specificity : divide D by (B+D)

Definition :   Specificity is the probability that a healthy patient (B+D) will have a negative test result (D).

Example :   A test has a specificity of 80% means that 20% of people without disease get a false positive (B) test result.

7.9.) <u>PREDICTIVE VALUES</u>

	patient is sick	patient is healthy
test result is positive	A	B
test result is negative	C	D

- Positive predictive value : divide A by (A+B)

- Definition: PPV is the probability that a patient with a positive test result (A+B) is really sick (A).

	patient is sick	patient is healthy
test result is positive	A	B
test result is negative	C	D

- Negative predictive value : divide D by (C+D)

- Definition: NPV is the probability that a patient with a negative test result (C+D) is really healthy (D).

 PPV is higher in populations with high prevalence!
NPV is higher in populations with low prevalence!

Specificity and sensitivity are independent of prevalence!

7.10.) <u>DEFENSE MECHANISMS</u>

Repression
Blocking of "dangerous" urges, feelings, thoughts from awareness.

Denial
Blocking of unacceptable information or perceptions from awareness.

Rationalization
Substituting an unacceptable motive for attitudes or behavior with acceptable motive.

Splitting
Maintaining a perception of others (or self) as all good or all bad

Projection
"You are acting like a teenager, not I !"

Reaction formation
You want to "kick his ass" and kiss it instead.

Isolation of affect
He talked about his sons's death calmly, without a sad expression in his face.

Displacement
You are angry with your boss and shout at your kids and husband instead.

Undoing
"Magic", like knocking on wood etc.

Transference
Unconscious tendency of patient to respond to the therapist as if he/she were someone else.

Countertransference
Unconscious tendency of therapist to respond to the patient as if he/she were someone else.

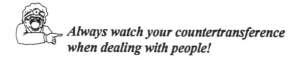 *Always watch your countertransference when dealing with people!*

258

7.11.) <u>CLINICAL TRIALS</u>

Retrospective case study. Useful for study of rare diseases

Cross-sectional survey. Association of two or more variables at a single point in time.
Example : Association between intravenous drug abuse and AIDS.

Observational cohort. Prospective or retrospective study to estimate incidence of disease in groups with different exposures

Randomized clinical trial. "State of the art" test to evaluate new drugs.

Chi square test. Analysis of categorical data distribution.
Example : Two groups of patients with rheumatoid arthritis are given either drug or placebo. Condition after treatment will be rated "improved", "same", or "worsened".

Paired Student's t-test. Each patient serves as its own control.
Example : Patients with hypertension are treated with placebo and drug in a "cross-over" design.

Correlation coefficient. Test of degree of association between two variables.
Example : Blood pressure and body Na^+ content are measured in cross-sectional study of patients.

Analysis of variance. Determine how several independent variables affect one dependent variable.
Example : Effect of race, sex and income on incidence of myocardial infarction.

Analysis of covariance. Determine how several independent variables affect one dependent variable and controlling for other variables.
Example : Assessment of effect of drug versus placebo in two groups of patients taking pretreatment blood pressure into account.

Factor analysis. Method to reduce many interrelated variables to few relatively independent factors.
Example : analysis of questionnaire that was originally designed to assess depression, anxiety, anger and pain.

ABBREVIATIONS

AA	amyloid associated protein
Ab	antibodies
ACh	acetylcholine
ADHD	attention deficit hyperactivity disorder
AFP	alpha fetoprotein
AL	amyloid light chains
ALA	aminolevulinate
ANA	antinuclear antibodies
AP	action potential
ASD	atrial septal defect
ARDS	acute resp. distress syndrome
a/w	associated with
BP	blood pressure
CA	carcinoma
CEA	carcinoembryonic antigen
CoA	coenzyme A
COPD	chronic obstructive pulmonary disease
CSF	cerebrospinal fluid
CNS	central nervous system
DES	diethylstilbestrol
DIC	disseminated intravascular coagulation
DOC	drug of choice
ds	double stranded
Dx	differential diagnosis
EBV	Epstein-Barr virus
ECV	extracellular volume
EEE	eastern equine encephalitis
EM	electron microscopy
G6PD	glucose-6-phosphate dehydrogenase
GABA	gamma-aminobutyrate
GBM	glomerular basement membrane
GH	growth hormone
GI	gastrointestinal
GN	glomerulonephritis
HCG	human chorionic gonadotropin
IDDM	insulin dependent diabetes mellitus
JGA	juxtaglomerular apparatus

LSD	lysergic acid diethylamide
MAC	minimal alveolar concentration
MAO	monoamine oxidase
MHC	major histocompatability complex
MI	myocardial infarction
MIF	Müllerian inhibiting factor
MLC	myosin light chain
MODY	maturaty onset diabetes of the young
NIDDM	non insulin dependent diabetes mellitus
NSAID	nonsteroidal antiinflammatory drug
PAH	p-aminohippurate
PAS	periodic acid Schiff reagant
PCP	phencyclidine
PDA	patent ductus arteriosus
PDE	phosphodiesterase
PG	prostaglandin
PMN	polymorph nuclear leukocyte
PT	prothrombin time
PTT	partial thromboplastin time
RBC	red blood cells
RSV	respiratory syncytial virus
Rx	treatment
SLE	systemic lupus erythematosus
ss	single stranded
SSPE	subacute sclerosing panencephalitis
TCA	tricyclic antidepressants
THC	tetrahydrocannabinol
TIA	transient ischemic attack
TPA	tissue plasminogen activator
TRAP	tartrate resistant alkaline phosphatase
TT	thrombin time
UTI	urinary tract infection
VD	venereal disease
VDRL	Venereal Disease Research Laboratory
VSD	ventricular septal defect
VZV	varicella zoster virus
WEE	western equine encephalitis